D1274389

LOW-FODMAP DIET COOKBOOK FOR BEGINNERS

Neutralize Scientifically the Enemies of the Sensitive Gut to Trot Through Quick and Tasty IBS Friendly Recipes | Rediscover Yourself Without Abdominal Pain with a 1000-Day Meal Plan for Bowel Relief

SARAH ROSLIN

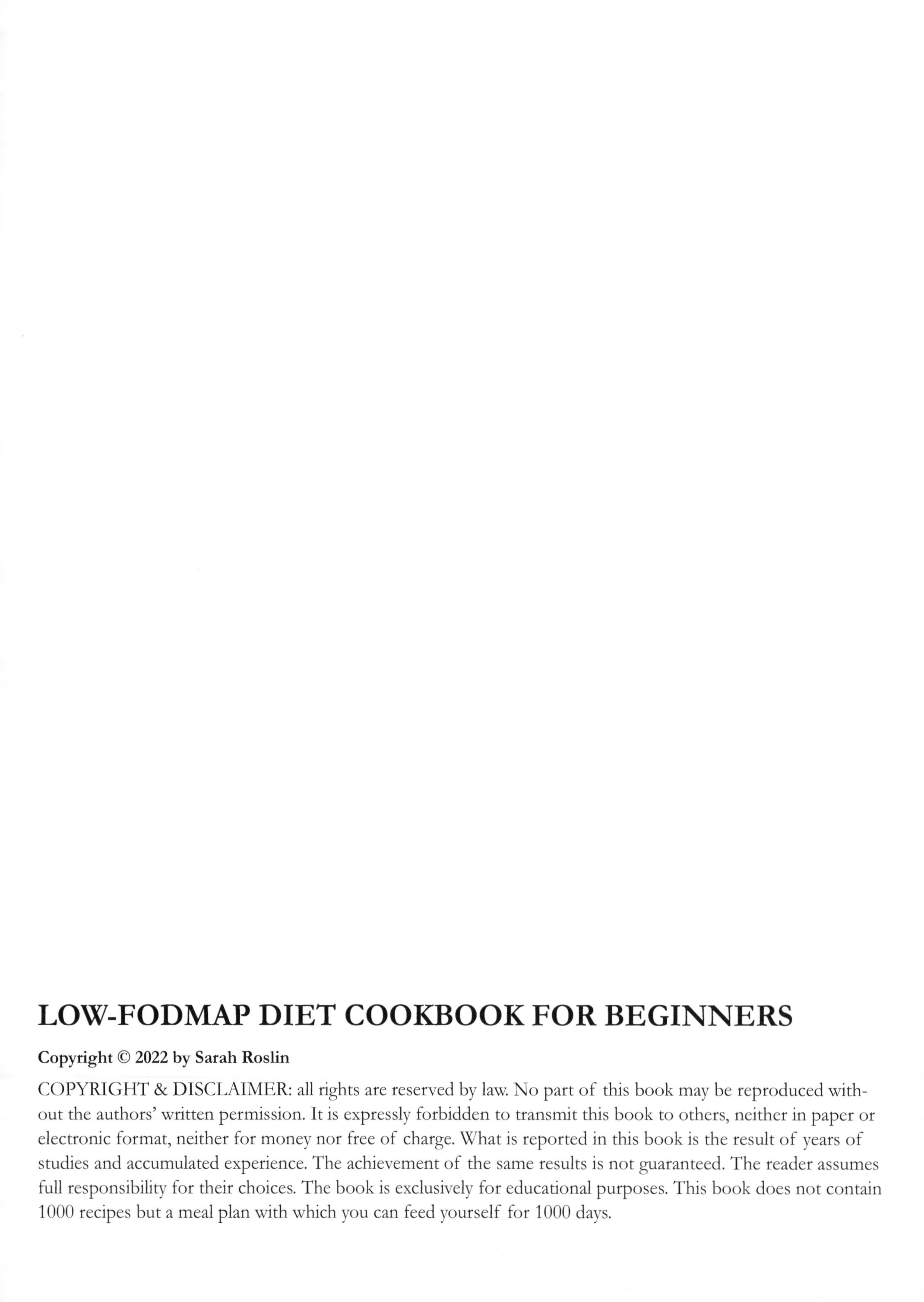

LOW-FODMAP DIET COOKBOOK FOR BEGINNERS

CONTENTS

INTRODUCTION

What is Low-FODMAP diet?

For the treatment of irritable bowel syndrome, specialists typically urge patients to adhere to the low-FODMAP diet, which contains few fermentable carbs (IBS)

The most typical digestive ailment in the U.S. is IBS. Food is often a common cause for symptoms like stomach pain and bloating for many persons with this condition.

These short-chain carbohydrates are osmotically active, which means that even if they are not digested, they force water into your digestive tract.

Furthermore, because they can't be digested, your gut bacteria ferment them, which results in more short-chain fatty acid and gas generation.

FODMAPs are well known for causing symptoms of the digestive system such as gas, bloating, stomach pain, and abnormal bowel habits like constipation, diarrhea, or a combination of both.

In fact, over 60% of IBS sufferers claim that these carbohydrates may either cause or aggravate their symptoms.

A wide variety of foods contain FODMAPs in various levels. Some foods only contain one kind, while others have a variety. The four classes of FODMAPs' main dietary sources are :

- **Oligosaccharides:** Wheat, rye, almonds, legumes, artichokes, garlic, and onion
- **Disaccharides:** Milk, yoghurt, soft cheese, ice cream, buttermilk, condensed milk, and whipped cream, all of which contain lactose.
- **Monosaccharides:** Mangoes Apples, watermelons and are examples of foods high in fructose. Other sweeteners high in fructose .
- **Polyols:** Xylitol and isomalt are low-calorie sweeteners that can be found in products like sugar-free gum and Mannitol. Mannitol and sorbitol can be found in apples, pears, cauliflower, stone fruits, mushrooms, and snow peas.

What is IBS

Irritable bowel syndrome is a condition that affects the large intestine (IBS). Some of the symptoms and warning indications include cramps, diarrhea, bloating, gas, and constipation. IBS is a chronic condition that needs ongoing care.

Only a small portion of IBS patients have severe symptoms and signs. Some people can alter their nutrition, manner of life, and other factors to manage their symptoms.

IBS signs and symptoms might vary, but they often last for a long time. The most prevalent examples are:

1. stomach pain that results from a bowel movement, such as cramping or bloating
2. changes in the appearance of bowel motions
3. changes in your bowel motions' frequency
4. Additional symptoms that are usually related include bloating, extra gas, or mucus in the stool.

Food and drinks to avoid in this diet

The following is a list of typical foods to stay away from, particularly if you have IBS:

Certain vegetables

- Leeks
- Sweet corn
- Brussels sprouts
- Mushrooms
- Cauliflower
- Snow peas
- Asparagus
- Cassava
- Choko
- Beetroot
- Celery -greater than 5cm of stalk
- Artichokes
- Black eyed peas
- Onions
- Butter beans
- Garlic

Fruits

- Apricots
- Nectarines
- Plums
- Watermelon
- Peaches
- Prunes
- Mangoes
- Pomegranate
- Prunes
- Raisins - over 1 tbsp / 13g
- Dates
- Feijoa
- Figs
- Goji berries
- Grapefruit - over 80g
- Guava, unripe
- Lychee
- Cherries
- Currants
- Blackberries
- Apples
- Pears
- Avocado

lentils and beans

- Pasta
- Cereals
- Rye and wheat
- Cracker Barrel
- Pizzerias
- Bread

Dairy Products

- Ice cream
- Pudding
- Cottage cheese
- Milk
- Yogurt
- Soft cheese
- Custard

Sugar Substitutes

- Sorbitol
- Xylitol
- Agave nectar
- High fructose corn syrup
- Maltitol
- Honey

Drinks

- Coconut water
- Sports drinks
- Alcohol
- Black tea with added soy milk
- Chai tea, strong
- Dandelion tea, strong
- Fennel tea
- Chamomile tea
- Herbal tea, strong
- Oolong tea

Condiments, Dips, Sweets, Sweeteners and Spreads

- Honey
- Jam, mixed berries
- Jam, strawberry, if contains HFCS
- Molasses
- Pesto sauce
- Quince paste
- Gravy, if it contains onion
- High fructose corn syrup (HFCS)
- Hummus
- Agave
- Caviar dip
- Fructose
- Fruit bar

Pros & Cons of this diet

Relief of Symptoms

The 95% of those eliminated found that a low FODMAP diet reduced or completely eliminate the most distressing gastrointestinal symptoms, such as bloating, discomfort, gas, and loose stools.

IBS can be subtyped based on in what way frequently or infrequently constipation or diarrhea occur. The four types of Constipation, diarrhea , mixed IBS, and IBS-U are the four types of IBS (neither). All of these subtypes have successfully experienced symptom reduction with low FODMAP.

Remember that compared to the other two types, IBS-M and IBS-U are far less common. Statistical analysis in these groups is therefore tricky. Low FODMAP diet's benefits for those with IBS-M and IBS-U have not been compared to the more common kinds of IBS..

Long-Term Comfort

Long-term reductions in IBS symptoms have been linked to completing the low FODMAP diet's three phases. In one study, 60 percent of IBS sufferers said their symptoms had improved "satisfactorily" a year after beginning the reduced FODMAP diet approach

Unfortunately, not even all long-term relief strategies improved the situation. Followers of the low-FOdmap diet missed the same number of days from work and visited the doctor at rates similar to those of individuals who ate their "normal" diets.

Even though more than half of the people who consume low-FODMAP foods say they feel better as a result, this diet is not a panacea.

Fewer histamines

A potent inflammatory signal are histamines. Histamines is implicated in allergy reactions and other immunological responses; whereas some foods directly contain it, others may cause an increase in histamines release

A reduced FODMAP diet for three weeks (21 days) led to an eight-fold reduction in urine histamines in one clinical research

Improved standard of living

In addition to lowering inflammation and its associated symptoms, the low FODMAP diet may improve various quality of life metrics in IBS patients. People with IBS who ate low-FODMAP reported

- Fewer feelings of anxiety, despair
- Less fatigue-related sensations
- Improved body image and less distress
- Less attention to health issues
- Heightened liveliness

Cons of this diet

Deficiencies in nutrients

FODMAP-rich foods frequently contain high levels of minerals and vitamins. Negligent risk of getting vitamin D, calcium, iron, zinc, and folate deficiency-related health problems.

Due to the large number of food categories that are excluded during the initial phase of the diet, this stage is the most hazardous, but it should only last a short time. Phases 2 and 3 won't be affected by nutrient deficits if you consult with a qualified nutritionist.

Balanced Gut Flora

Nutrient-rich food is necessary for healthy gut flora to survive and flourish. Some beneficial bacteria, such as Bifidobacteria, which feed on FODMAPs, might experience a reduction in population on a low-FODMAP diet.

When helpful bacteria degrade small carbohydrate molecules in the stomach, short-chain fatty acids (SCFAs), such as butyrate, are produced. These ,in turn, give the big intestine's lining cells sustenance. For optimal gut health, some FODMAPs may be necessary.

If you do not have IBS, a low-FODMAP diet, may be harmful to your gut flora. This is one of the reasons it's essential to consult a doctor before starting the diet.

Costly

People following a stringent FODMAP diet may need to spend more money on costlier alternatives, such as exotic fruits and "pseudo-cereals," to prevent nutritional deficits (such as amaranth, quinoa, and buckwheat)

Only people with higher socioeconomic status can successfully follow a low-FODMAP diet because these fees are typically not covered by health insurance.

Healthy Low-FODMAP Diet Secrets

1. Create a meal with fewer FODMAPs

Making dinner decisions will be easier if you have a daily meal plan or even a stack of recipes you enjoy.

Meal planning, meal preparation, and even research on Low FODMAP meals at nearby restaurants are all options.

2. THE KEY TO THIS WHOLE DIET IS PORTION SIZE.

Low-FODMAP is always uses a serving.. I am aware that this can be challenging. In the case of fruits and vegetables, it could be challenging to limit oneself to 10 raspberries or a half cup of cantaloupe. However, use caution and be aware of how much you take from the bowl to avoid consuming too much of that substance.

3. FODMAPs are found in garlic and onion powder.

These may also be present in blended spices (read the labels). Keep to low-FODMAP seasonings; there are many options available. My low-FODMAP Happy Spices Seasoning Blends might be your favorite (Taco, Steak ,and Italian).

4. FODMAPs are frequently concealed in "natural" flavors in savory soups, broths, and frozen foods.

Assume that these contain onion and garlic, and decide against including many of these seasonings in a meal. FODMAP is not low!

5. FODMAPs can dissolve in water but not in fat.

This means that even if you prepare soup with onion and then remove the onion, the soup will still contain onion FODMAPs. Don't consume it! Since FODMAPs are not fat-soluble, it is okay to use onion-infused oils; just the flavor will endure.

6. FODMAPs may be present in beverages.

Chicory in coffee is not low-FODMAP. Intense black, oolong, dandelion, chamomile, and fennel teas are not low-FODMAP. The absence of net carbs does not necessarily imply the absence of FODMAPs.

CHAPTER 1

FAQ

1. How can I add flavor to food without onion or garlic?

Due to their high FODMAP fructan content, garlic and onions are not recommended for those following the low FODMAP diet. Onions and garlic can, however, be used to enhance the flavor of your food.

Using garlic-infused oil is a fantastic approach to restoring flavor to your food as FODMAPs are not soluble in oil. To accomplish this, sauté whole pieces of unchopped, unmashed garlic in oil for one to two minutes to bring out the flavor of the oil. After that, take out and throw away the garlic because the clove itself still contains a lot of FODMAPs.

2. Which cheeses contain FODMAPs?

The FODMAP found in many dairy products is known by the term lactose. Hard cheeses and other matured or "ripened" cheeses, such feta cheese ,camembert, and brie, typically contain little or no lactose. Examples of cheeses having a mild lactose level include halloumi cheese, cream cheese, and ricotta cheese.

3. Do goods designated as fructose friendly meet the same standards?

No, the only goods that have complied with the requirements of the certified trademark and been given ACCC approval are FODMAP Friendly certified.

4. On a low FODMAP diet, what foods are permitted?

Foods that are low in FODMAPs include oats, millets, gluten-free items, strawberries, cottage cheese, lactose-free milk, broccoli, cottage cheese, eggplant, kiwifruit, and nuts like walnuts and almonds and chicken, salmon,

5. How does a low-FODMAPS diet function?

A low-FODMAP diet entails three stages of elimination:

You first give up eating particular foods (high FODMAP foods).

You then gradually reintroduce them to determine which ones are problematic.

Once you know which meals trigger your symptoms, you can limit or avoid them while still enjoying in all other foods without concern.

Veloso says, "We recommend only following the elimination portion of the diet for two to six weeks." This lessens your symptoms and, if you have SIBO, it may aid in lowering excessively high amounts of gut bacteria. After that, you can gradually reintroduce one high FODMAP food into your diet every three days to check for side effects. Avoid a particular high-FODMAP food if it produces symptoms.

6. I get irritable bowel syndrome symptoms after eating wheat. Should I start the low FODMAP diet?

Like celiac disease, irritable bowel syndrome symptoms include abdominal bloating, increased wind, stomach pain, diarrhea, constipation, or a mix of both. Wheat isa problematic food for both the gluten-free and low-FODMAP diets, it is vital to know. Before making dietary changes, it is imperative to discuss being tested for celiac disease with your doctor. Your doctor can arrange blood tests and even a gastroscopy to check for celiac disease, but you must still eat gluten for these to be effective. The low-FODMAP diet may be effective treatment if celiac disease is not present. Consult with your doctor and a qualified nutritionist to understand the low FODMAP diet's two phases as quickly and efficiently as possible.

7. Regarding spelling, I'm not sure. Despite some information to the contrary, spelt-based items can be found with the FODMAP Friendly badge. Would you kindly elaborate?

While FODMAPs are present in spelt, they are far less prevalent than in ordinary wheat. Since the number of FODMAPs in the Whole berry muffins and cookies, which use spelt flour rather than standard wheat flour, has been tested and found to be minimal, these goods can use the FODMAP Friendly label. The FODMAP Friendly label is a wonderful way to identify goods that have been tested to be low FODMAP per Sufficient for because other products containing spelt might not be. Please be aware that spelt contains gluten and is not ideal for those who follow a gluten-free diet.

8. How is this product appropriate for someone like myself who is lactose intolerant but has been taught that hard cheese can have the FODMAP Friendly emblem on it?

Aged cheeses either have almost no lactose or only a tiny amount that usually doesn't bother most people. Hard cheeses have been put through scientific testing to ensure they meet the FODMAP friendly requirements.

9. Are meats low in FODMAPs?

As they contain little to no carbohydrates, animal protein sources such meat, fowl, fish, and eggs are often low in FODMAPs. However, watch out for components used in the preparation of these foods that may be high in FODMAPs, such as bread crumbs, onions, garlic, marinades, sauces, and gravies. As they contain little to no carbohydrates, animal protein sources such meat, fowl, fish, and eggs are often low in FODMAPs.

10. Which foods should you avoid if you have IBS?

Fermentable Oligo-, Di-, Monosaccharides, and Polyols (FODMAPs)-containing foods can make IBS symptoms worse. Wheat, garlic, onion, apple, cow's milk, fermented vegetables, pistachios, cashews, and a number of other foods are examples.

CHAPTER 2

LOW FODMAP DIET APP

Monash University's mobile app, titled "Monash University Low FODMAP Diet App" in the Android and iPhone app stores, is a helpful resource for studying FODMAP (fermentable oligosaccharides, disaccharides, monosaccharides, and polyols) foods. Using a traffic light system to identify foods based on portion size helps reduce confusion over the correct number of servings. The app contains information about irritable bowel syndrome, recipes, and meal ideas. Monash offers Low FODMAP certification for foods, goods, recipes, and online training

PLAY STORE

APPSTORE

LEGEND

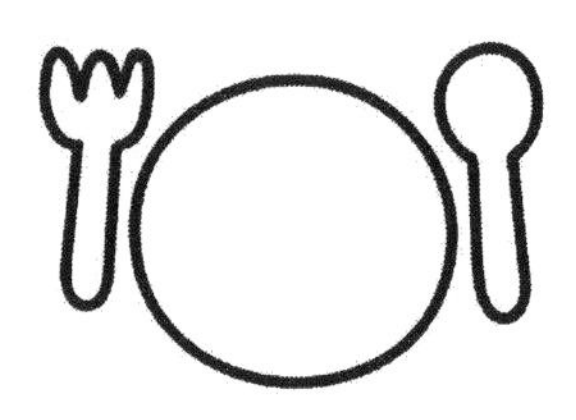

Serves Plate

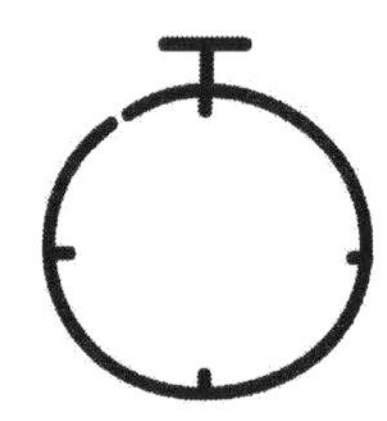

Preparation Time Clock

Cooking Time Pot

Nutrition Facts

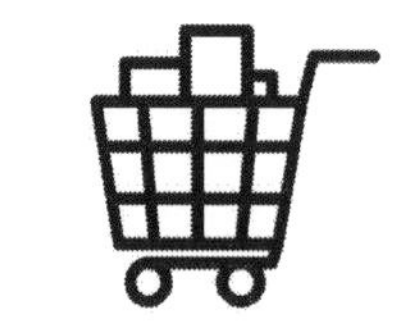

Ingredients Full Cart

Procedure Book

Calories

Total Fat

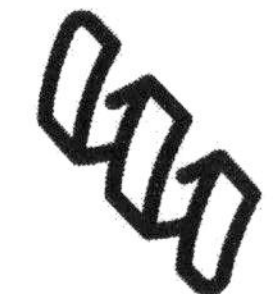

Protien

Total Carbohydrate

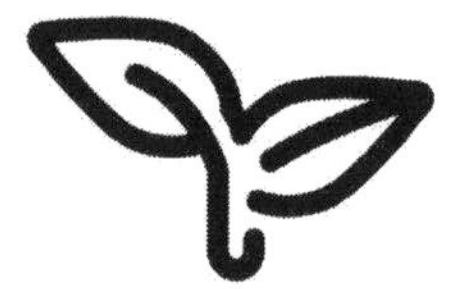

Dietary Fiber

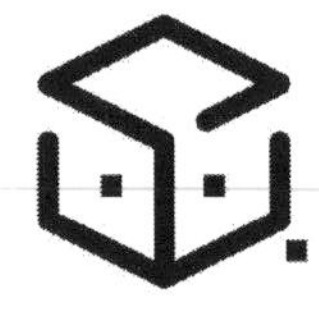

Sugar

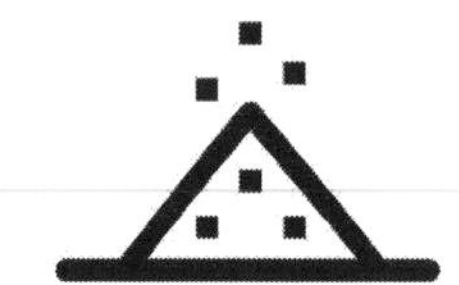

Sodium

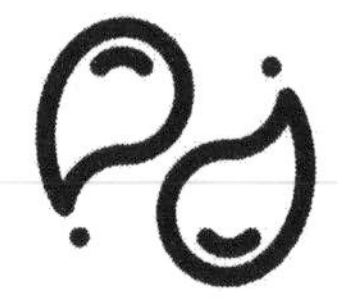

Cholesterol

Total Energy

CHAPTER 3

BREAKFAST RECIPES

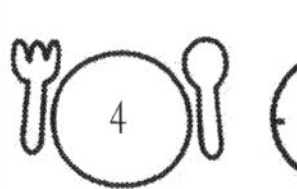 4 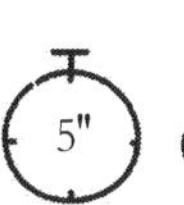 5"  25"

3.1 Quinoa Porridge

 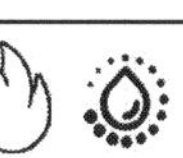 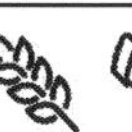 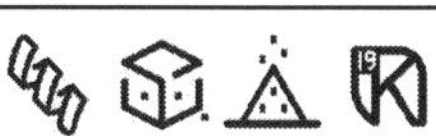 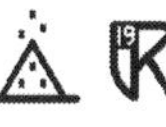

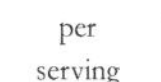 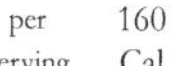

per serving | 160 Cal | 9.7g | 15.8g | 4g | 1.1g | 213 mg

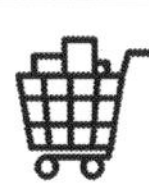

- Brazil nuts ¼ cup
- Water 1 ¼ cups
- Quinoa ½ cup
- Cinnamon ½ teaspoon
- Coconut milk ½ cup
- taste-tested amounts of Stevia

1. Place the quinoa and water in a medium saucepan and heat over high heat until it boils. As soon as it starts to boil, lower the heat to low and cover the pot.
2. It takes 25 to 30 minutes to cook quinoa to a soft consistency. Dispose of any leftover water by draining it. Add the coconut milk, cinnamon, and brazil nuts after five minutes. Try it out.

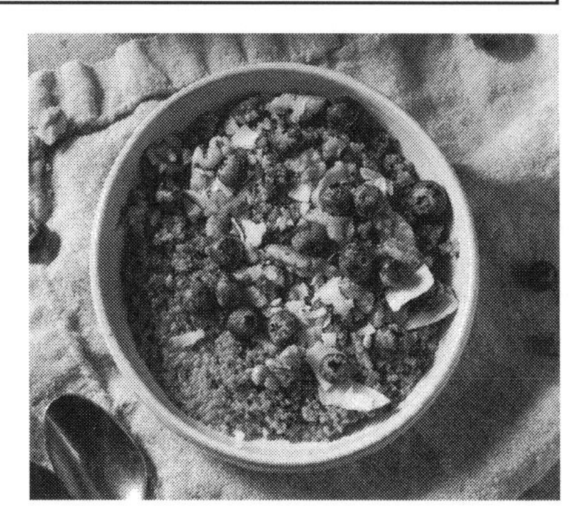

Storage:
The porridge can be frozen for up to 3 months maintained in the refrigerator for up to 5 days.

Reheat:
Reheat the porridge in the microwave before eating.

3.2 Pancakes with strawberries

	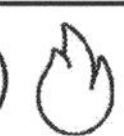	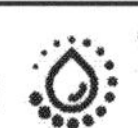	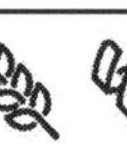	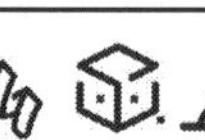	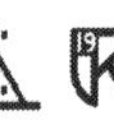
per serving	129 Cal	4.2g	17.8	5.8g 2.2g	226 mg

- Baking powder, -1/2 tsp.
- Salt, -1/4 tsp.
- Strawberries, -1 cup
- Oats,- 1 cup
- Unripe bananas, mashed -1/4 cup
- Vanilla essence, -1/2 tsp.
- Baking soda, -1/4 tsp.
- Water-1 tbsp.
- Eggs, -2
- Walnut flour, - 2 tbsp

1. Slice or cut the strawberries into thirds.
2. To create a homogeneous batter, combine the egg, raw oats, mashed banana, baking powder, baking soda, salt, vanilla essence, walnut flour, and water.
3. Fold the strawberries into the mixture after pouring it into a small bowl.
4. Warm up a medium nonstick pot. Place 1/4 or 1/2 of the batter in the center of the pan, cover it with the lid, and As soon as possible, lower the heat. the batter is cooked until the top is completely dry. Cook the second side till golden brown by flipping it over. Continue with the remaining batter.
5. Sufficient for and . Enjoy.

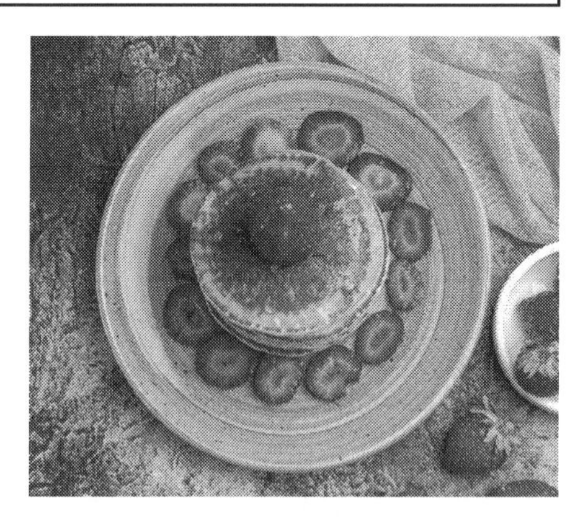

Storage:
Put the pancakes in a freezer-safe container for storage (ziploc bag, empty bread bag, or tupperware).

Reheat:
Larger batches of pancakes can be reheated as follows: 350 degrees Fahrenheit in the oven.

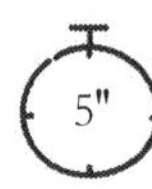

3.3 Prepared scrambled eggs with cheese.

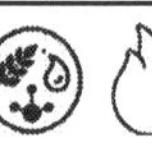	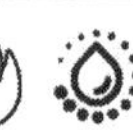	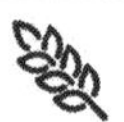	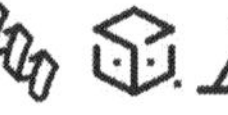	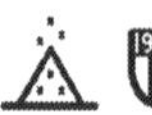	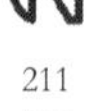
per serving	314 Cal	20g	13.8g	20g 3.8g	211 mg

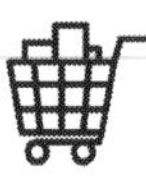

- Salt to taste
- Gluten-free bread, -2 slices
- Oil, - 1 tsp.
- Eggs, -4
- Feta cheese, -1/2 cup

1. Pour oil into a frying pan and turn it on to heat.
2. With a fork, quickly beat the eggs after breaking them into a bowl.
3. Prepare the cheese by grating it.
4. In the frying pan, pour the beaten eggs.
5. cheese is layered on top.
6. As soon as the eggs almost instantly start to firm, "pull" them in from the side to the center with a spatula.
7. Pulling in should be repeated multiple times.
8. You're finished when the egg has no more "watery" components. Remove from fire immediately and place on plate, ideally on top of some delicious, hot, unbuttered bread.
9. As desired, add salt.

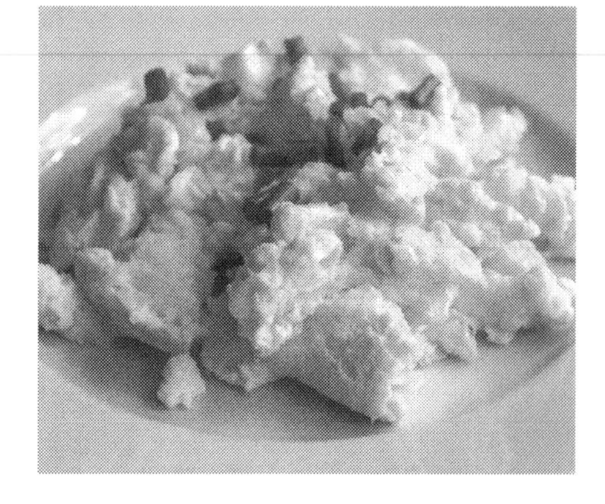

Storage:
They should be cooled quickly and evenly in a shallow container before being kept in the refrigerator at 40°F (4°C) or below. Eat any leftover eggs within 3–4 days

Reheat:
Eggs are tastiest when eaten right away, but you may gently reheat them in a low oven or a nonstick skillet.

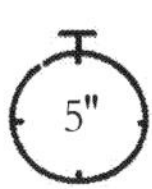

3.4 Breakfast Egg Muffins

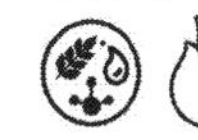
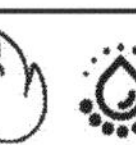
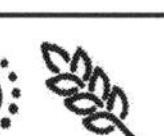
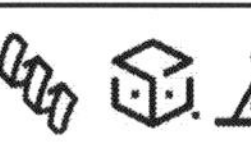
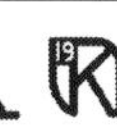

per serving	256 Cal	17.2g	5.8g	20.1g	3.3g	327 mg

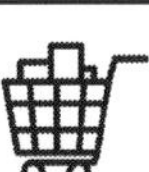

- 12 eggs
- 1 cup kale
- ½ cup feta cheese
- ¼ tsp salt
- 1 bell pepper,

1. Set the oven's temperature to 200 C/ 390 F.
2. Bell peppers should be cleaned, diced, and added to a sizable mixing bowl.
3. Additionally, add the washed, excellently cut kale to the bowl.
4. Salt and eggs are added. Mix well. Mix in the cheese with the batter..
5. Using baking paper or a brush, grease the muffin tin with oil and then pour the egg mixture into the muffin holes in a uniform layer..
6. The tops should feel firm to the touch after 20 minutes in the oven.

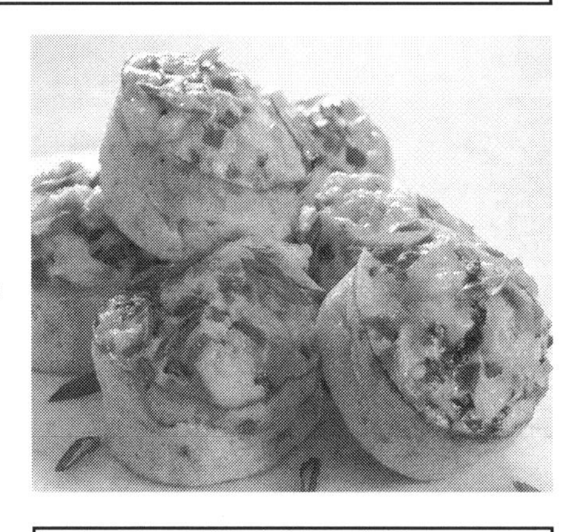

Storage:
Up to three months of frozen muffin storage are possible.

Reheat:
Reheat for an hour or until hot while wrapped in foil at 300 °F (150 °C). Remove the packaging and put the pudding in the original mould to reheat on the stove. Wrap tightly

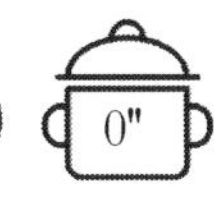

3.5 Flax Seed Pudding

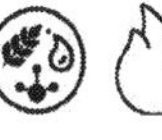

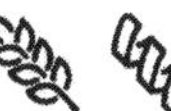
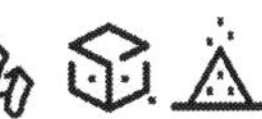
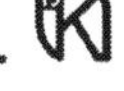

per serving	483 Cal	43.2g	18.7g	7.3g	8.8g	604 mg

- Vanilla extract-4 tbsp
- Flax seeds -8 tbsp.
- Strawberries (cut in halves) – 2 cups
- Pecan – 4 tbsp.
- Stevia -1/4 tsp
- Salt- 1/4 tsp.
- Coconut milk -2 cups

1. A small pot with the following ingredients is heated over medium heat: coconut milk, stevia, vanilla extract, and salt. As soon as the liquid reaches a rolling boil, remove off the fire.
2. Pour the coconut milk and flax seed mixture into a larger bowl. Until all of the seeds are evenly in contact with the liquid, stir continuously. Cover and let the food sit in the refrigerator for 12 hours or overnight.
3. Before serving, top the flax pudding with pecans and strawberries.

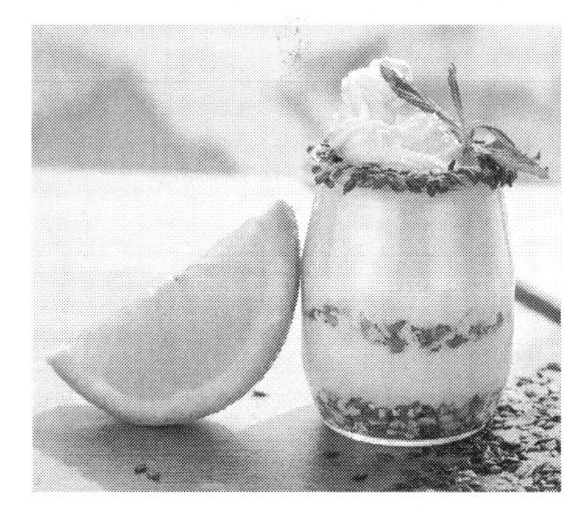

Storage:
To protect it, place it in an sealed dish and wrap it in plastic. Keep refrigerated for a week maximum.

Reheat:
Reheat for an hour or until hot while wrapped in foil at 300 °F (150 °C). Remove the packaging and put the pudding in the original mould to reheat on the stove. Wrap tightly

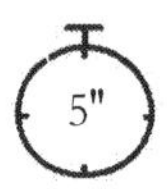

3.6 Buckwheat Breakfast Porridge

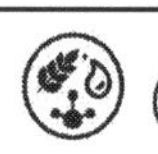 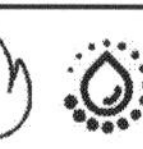 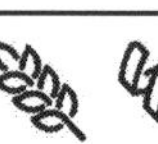 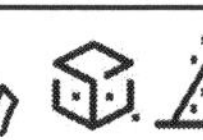 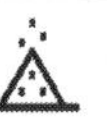

per serving	484 Cal	34.8g	41.5g	10.6g	5.9g	613 mg

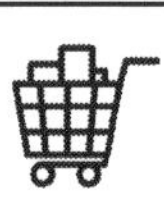

- Cinnamon – 1 tsp
- Buckwheat – 1 cup
- 1 pinch salt
- Walnut (chopped) -4 tbsp.
- Coconut milk – 2 cups
- Water- 1 cup,
- Strawberries, fresh -16 tbsp.

1. Use two parts liquid to one part buckwheat while cooking buckwheat. Thoroughly rinse the buckwheat. Buckwheat, water, and coconut milk must all be combined in a vessel. Bring up to a boil before lowering the heat. There is no need for a lid.
2. Salt, and cinnamon can now be added.
3. Slice the walnuts, and add them to the saucepan as well. Keep a few of each aside for garnish.
4. 20 minutes or so of simmering is usually sufficient to soften the buckwheat and absorb the liquid.
5. In the meantime, take a pan and add the strawberries. Using fresh ones will with a fork, slightly mash them. Let them cook until marmalade-like. That should take five minutes.
6. Take a bowl and put the buckwheat inside. More coconut milk should be added to your mixture. The strawberry sauce is now included. To finish it off, add a few extra pecans slices Enjoy!

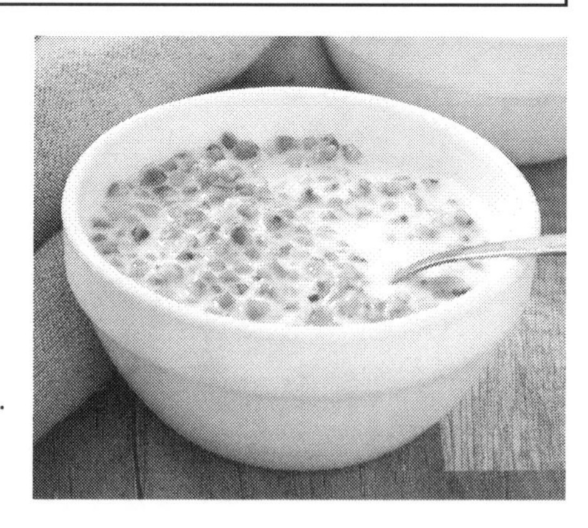

Storage:
The porridge can be frozen for up to 3 months or Keep refrigerated for a week maximum.

Reheat:
Reheat the porridge in the microwave before eating.

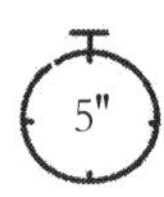

3.7 Tomato Omelet

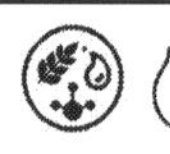 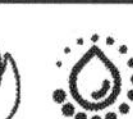 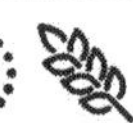 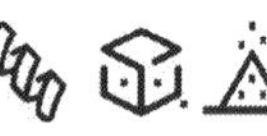  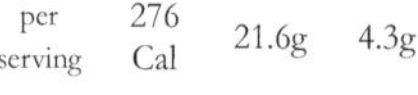 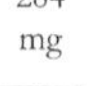

per serving	276 Cal	21.6g	4.3g	16.2g	3.5g	284 mg

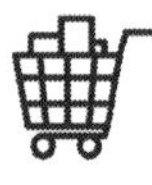

- Feta cheese -¾ cup
- Salt (to taste)
- Olive oil -4 tsp.
- Tomato -1 medium
- Eggs -8
- Basil, fresh -1 cup

1. Wash the tomatoes and, then slice them into small pieces.
2. The tomatoes should be fried for around 2 minutes in a pan with half the oil heated. Set separately. Utilize a tissue to wipe the pan.
3. Add the salt and cracked eggs to a bowl and whisk the mixture well..
4. In a pan, preferably Heat the remaining oil in a nonstick pan over low to medium heat. Utilize paper to lightly wipe the oil away (or an oil spray if you have it).
5. Mixture of eggs should be added to the pan..
6. The omelet should be fluffed using a spatula to avoid going to stick. As gaps are made, turn the pan so that the liquid fills them.
7. Give it about two minutes to fry, then
8. The crucial step is to add the tomatoes, basil, cheese, when the egg mixture is almost fully cooked but still has a tiny bit of runny egg left.
9. On top of the other half of the omelet, fold the empty half.
10. The heat from sealing the omelet will finish cooking the inside as you slide it onto a platter.

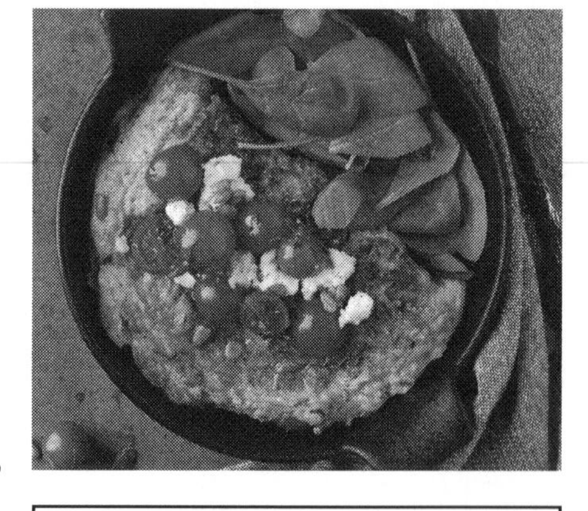

Storage:
In an airtight container, your omelet is safe to Preserve in the fridge for 3-4 days. Before putting them in the refrigerator, make sure to seal them up in an airtight bag or container. Ziplock bags work nicely for storing omelets. Better yet, you can freeze your omelet for up to 4 months.

Reheat:
For 1 to 1 1/2 minutes on high, microwave omelets covered until thoroughly heated.

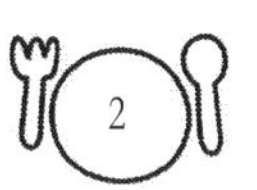 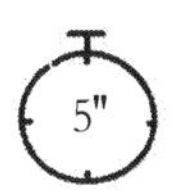 

2 5" 10"

3.8 Banana Egg Pancakes

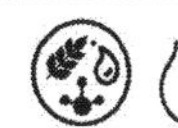 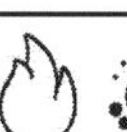 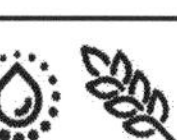 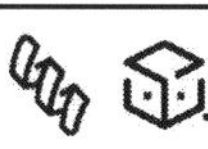 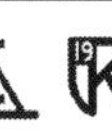

per serving	251 Cal	11.5g	27.6g	12.4g	15g	540 mg

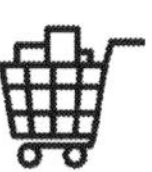

- 8 tbsp, mashed unripe banana
- ½ tsp Olive oil
- 4 eggs

1. To whisk eggs, simply use a fork. and include in the banana paste.
2. Gently fry using a small amount of hot oil over low to medium heat.
3. With a large spatula, flip the food halfway through cooking (approximately 4 minutes).

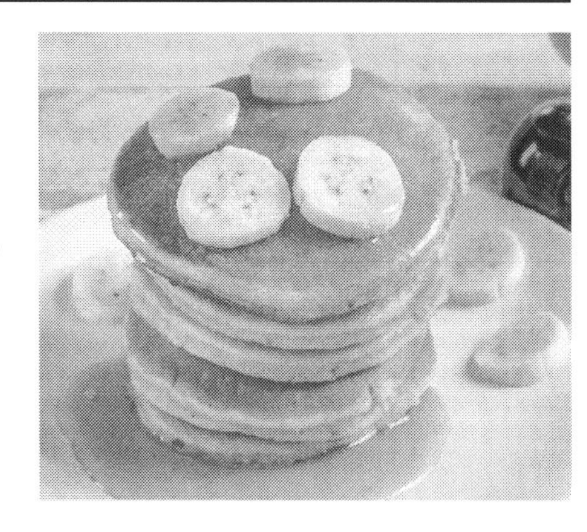

Storage:
Put the pancakes in a freezer-safe container for storage (ziploc bag, empty bread bag, or tupperware).

Reheat:
To reheat bigger batches of pancakes, a 350 degree Fahrenheit oven preheat. Put the pancakes Place them on a baking sheet in a single layer, then cover with foil.

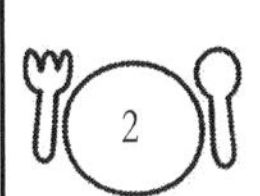 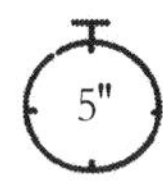 

2 5" 5"

3.9 Eggs in Cloud

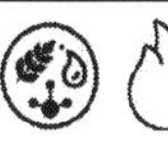  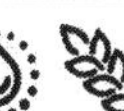 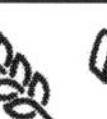  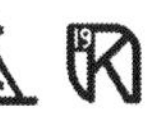 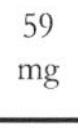

per serving	63 Cal	4.5g	0.3g	5.5g	0.3g	59 mg

- Two eggs
- a generous pinch of sea salt

1. Start the oven, first. Set a baking sheet to 450°F and cover it with parchment paper.
2. Carefully separate the egg whites from the yolks, being careful not to crack the yolks.
3. Place the In a stand mixer equipped with a whisk, combine egg whites and a pinch of salt. attachment. The egg whites should be whipped until stiff peaks form.
4. Evenly spread tiny clouds of the egg white mixture positioned on the lined baking sheet.
5. Bake the egg whites for 3 minutes with the baking sheet in the center of the oven.
6. Gently place one egg yolk on top of each cloud. three more minutes of baking.
7. Immediately Sufficient for the meal after taking it out of the oven.

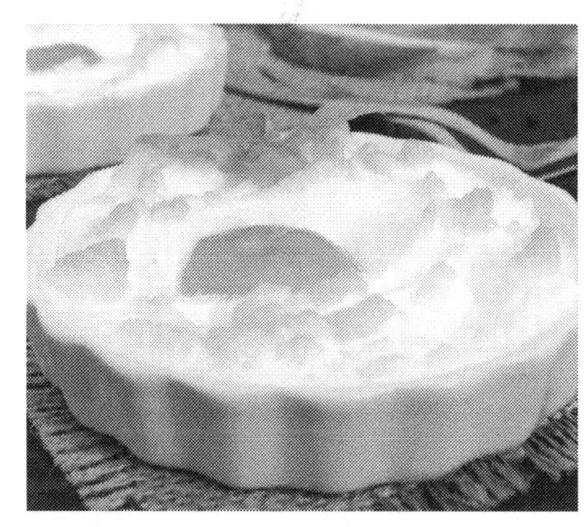

Storage:
They should be cooled quickly and evenly in a shallow container before being kept in the refrigerator at 40°F (4°C) or below. Eat any leftover eggs within 3–4 days

Reheat:
Eggs are tastiest when eaten right away, but you may gently reheat them in a low oven or a nonstick skillet.

 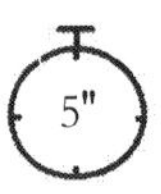 

8 | 5" | 20"

3.10 Baked Eggs in Kale and Tomato

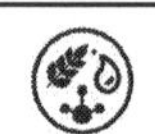 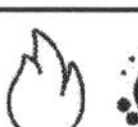  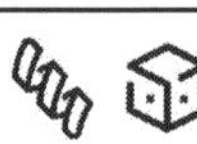 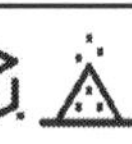 

per serving	169 Cal	10.9g	8.2g	10.7g	2.2g	401 mg

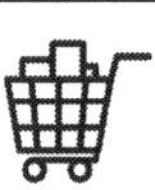

- 8 eggs
- 2 medium tomato
- 2 cups feta cheese
- 2 teaspoons of olive oil
- 2 cups basil (chopped)
- Salt
- 8 cups kale

1. Set the oven's temperature to 200 C (400 F).
2. Slice the tomatoes.
3. Combine the kale with the tomatoes.
4. Only the eggs should be set aside as you add and whisk everything else.
5. Wipe some olive oil all over the bowl(s) to grease them. Make wells in the center of the mixture in two small ovenproof basins (or one large one).
6. Fill the wells with the cracked eggs..
7. For 20 minutes, bake at 200 °C (400 °F).
8. Serve the eggs. When ready, remove the dish from the oven. No need to continue cooking.
9. Top with a further sprinkle of salt.
10. Have fun with nice,

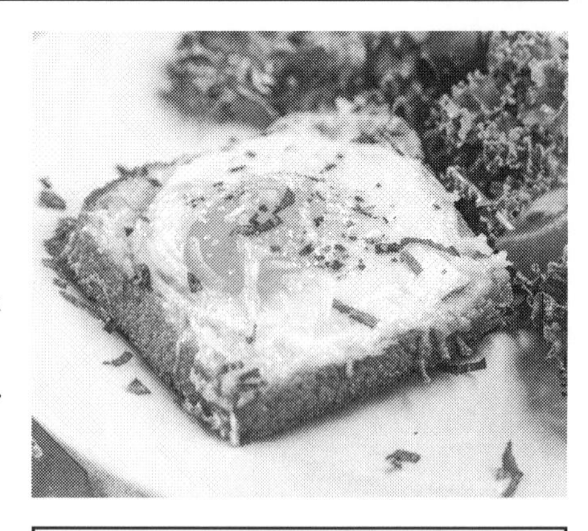

Storage:
They should be cooled quickly and evenly in a shallow container before being kept in the refrigerator at 40°F (4°C) or below. Eat any leftover eggs within 3–4 days

Reheat:
Eggs are tastiest when eaten right away, but you may gently reheat them in a low oven or a nonstick skillet.

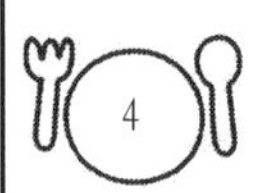 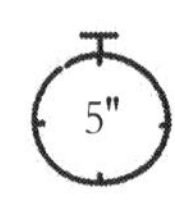 

4 | 5" | 20"

3.11 Sesame Breakfast Pudding

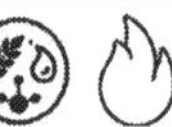 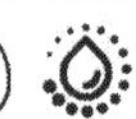 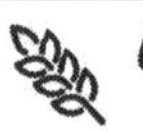 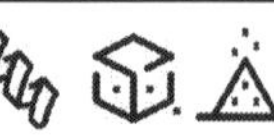 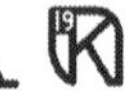

per serving	268 Cal	22.3	18.2g	4.3g	8.3g	381 mg

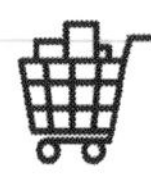

- 8 tbsp, of sesame seeds;
- 4 tiny unripe banana
- 4 tbsp, cacao powder
- 2 cups almond milk
- 4 tbsp, ground Macadamia nut
- 2 teaspoons stevia

1. 1. Use a fork to mash the banana in a bowl. After that, divide the mash between four glasses.
2. Now combine the milk, sesame seeds, and cacao powder in a bowl. Use a mixer (we use this immersion blender) to prevent cacao lumps. or an equivalent.
3. Over the banana mash, pour the mixture.
4. Finally, add grated Macadamia nut as a garnish. They can be grated using a food processor. Or simply use whole Macadamia nut as a garnish.
5. Place the pudding in the refrigerator for about eight hours. Enjoy!

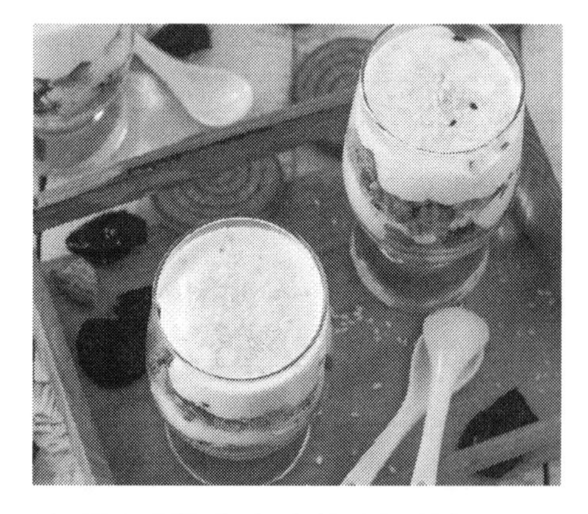

Storage:
The Pudding can be frozen for up to 3 months maintained in the maintained in the refrigerator for up to 5 days.

Reheat:
In the microwave just before eating, reheat the Pudding

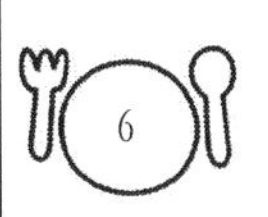
6
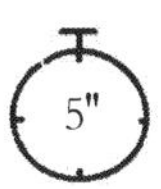
5"

15"

3.12 Egg muffins with quinoa

 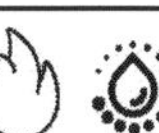 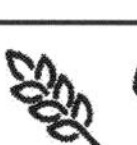 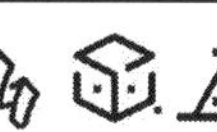 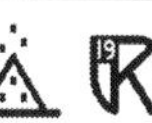

per serving	275 Cal	10.7g	31g	14.3g	2.6g		90g

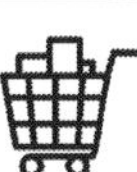

- 6 tbsp. grapes
- Quinoa cooked in 4 cups
- 1 tbsp. olive oil
- 8 eggs
- Salt to taste

1. Set the oven to 200 °C or 390 °F.
2. Eggs should be beaten in a big bowl.
3. Mashed the banana.
4. Add the sesame seed to the bowl with them. Add salt, cacao powder and banana.
5. Oil the muffin tin with a light brush.
6. Put the batter into the twelve muffin tins.
7. For 10 to 12 minutes, cook.
8. It's finished now! Enjoy.

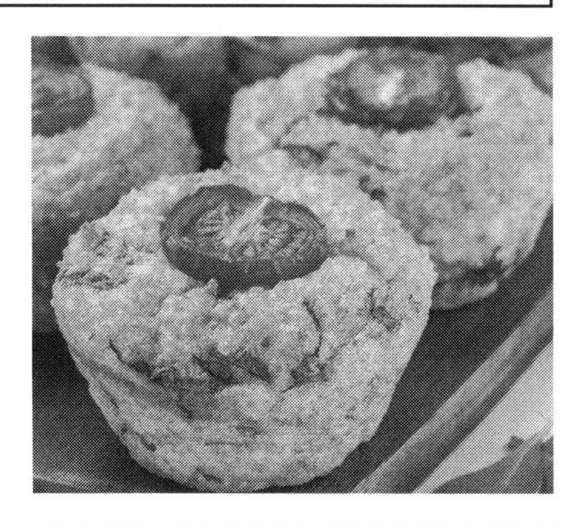

Storage:
Up to three months of frozen muffin storage are possible

Reheat:
Muffins can be heated in the microwave or regular oven as indicated, or they can be thoroughly defrosted at room temperature.

2
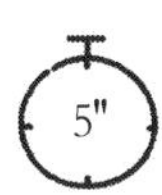
5"

0"

3.13 Overnight Oats

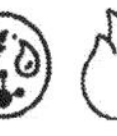 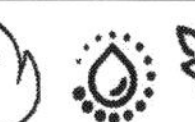 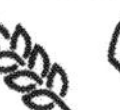 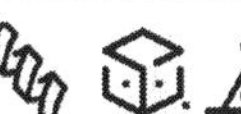 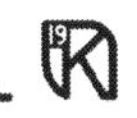

per serving	376 Cal	21g	30.1g	10g	4.1g		337 mg

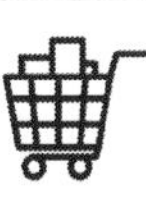

- Rolling oats, 1 cup
- 4 tsp flax seeds
- 1 cup strawberries,
- 2 tbsp. walnuts (chopped)
- 2 tsp stevia
- 1 cup coconut milk

1. Put the coconut milk, flax seeds, and oats in a jar. Stir everything thoroughly to combine it.
2. Then it is placed overnight in the refrigerator (or for at least six hours).
3. Add a little extra coconut milk the following morning to loosen the mixture.
4. The strawberries, stevia, and chopped walnuts can then be combined, and breakfast is ready!

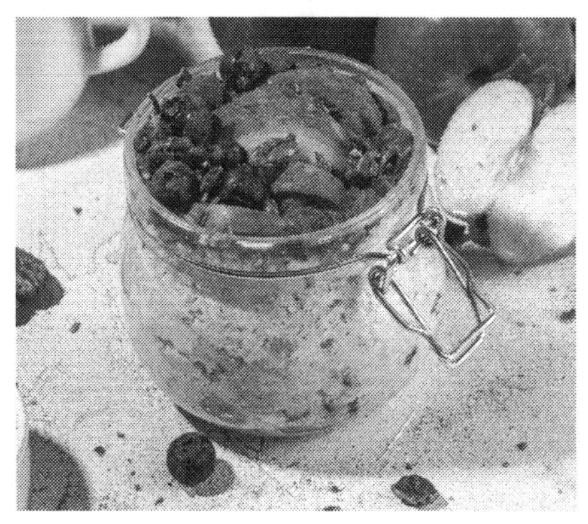

Storage:
The porridge can be frozen for up to 3 months or kept in the maintained in the refrigerator for up to 5 days.

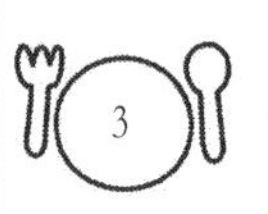

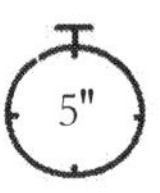

3.14 Peppers Scrambled Eggs

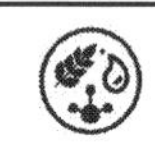 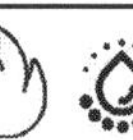 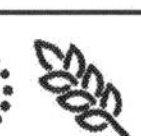 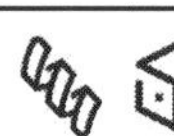 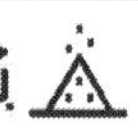 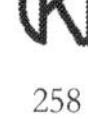

per serving	304 Cal	23.9g	6.8g	17g	5.2g	258 mg

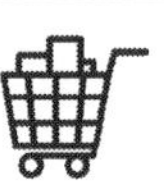

- Olive oil – 2tbsp.
- Green bell peppers, chopped - 2
- Eggs - 4
- Sea salt, fine – ¼ tsp.
- Feta cheese crumbles -1 cup
- Freshly chopped cilantro – 6 tbsp.

1. Warm the olive oil in a 10-inch, big, oil-filled skillet.
2. Including pepper and salt. Sauté for a few minutes, or until you're satisfied with the texture.
3. In the meantime, whisk the eggs in a small bowl.
4. Medium-low heat should be used. Cook the eggs in the skillet until just set after pouring them in, using a silicone spatula to move the eggs to the center as they cook beneath.
5. Add cheese, cilantro, to taste, enjoy.

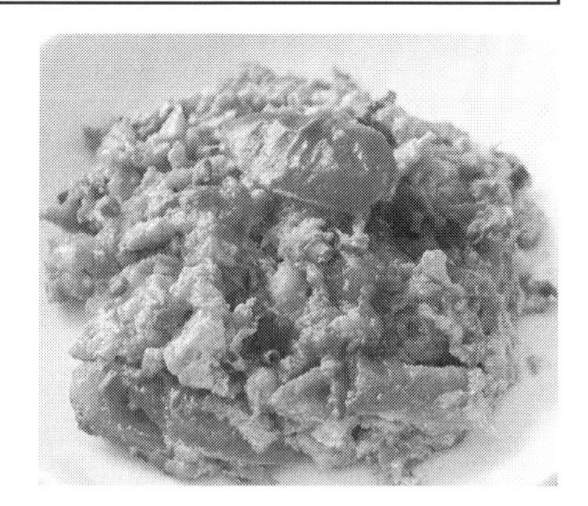

Storage:
They should be cooled quickly and evenly in a shallow container before being kept in the refrigerator at 40°F (4°C) or below. Eat any leftover eggs within 3–4 days

Reheat:
Eggs are tastiest when eaten right away, but you may gently reheat them in a low oven or a non-stick skillet.

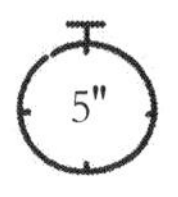

3.15 Flaxseed Flour Muffins

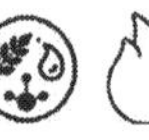 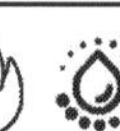 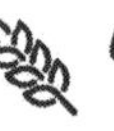 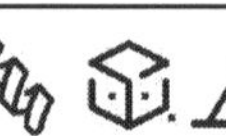 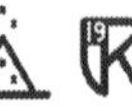 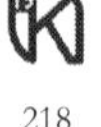

per serving	119 Cal	4.9g	14.8g	4.9g	7.1g	218 mg

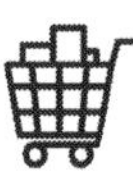

- 2 small unripe banana
- 2 eggs
- 1 tbsp. strawberries, chopped
- 1 tbsp. flaxseed flour
- salt to taste
- ¼ tsp cinnamon

1. Set the oven's temperature to 180 C/360 F.
2. Mash the banana in a bowl.
3. Additionally, crack the eggs into it. Add salt, cinnamon, strawberries, and flaxseed flour.
4. The mixture should be thoroughly forked.
5. Distribute the mixture into 2 ramekins or tiny bowls.
6. It is baked for 20 to 25 minutes in the oven.
7. Take pleasure in heat or cold.

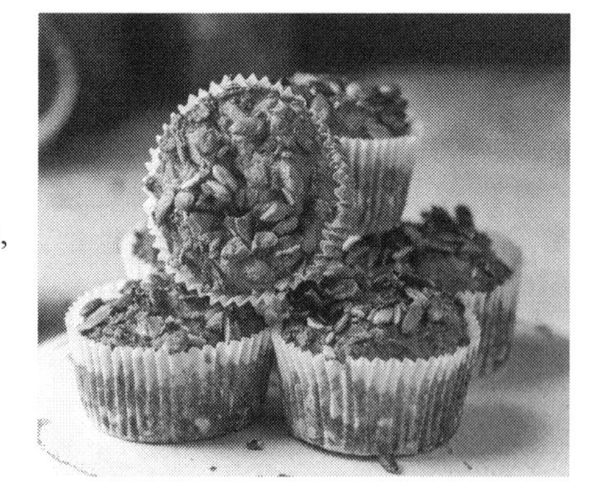

Storage:
Up to three months of frozen muffin storage are possible.

Reheat:
Muffins can be heated in the microwave or regular oven as indicated, or they can be thoroughly defrosted at room temperature.

CHAPTER 4

SALAD RECIPES

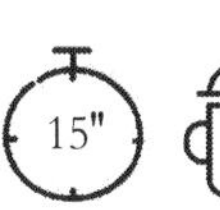

8 | 15" | 5"

4.1 Easy Kale Salad

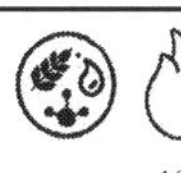
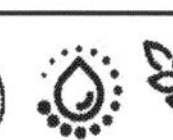
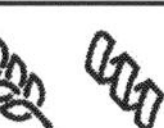
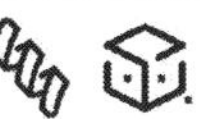
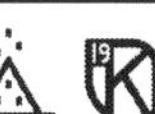
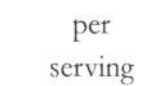
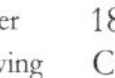
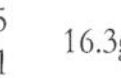
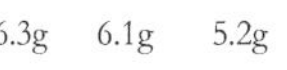
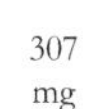

per serving	185 Cal	16.3g	6.1g	5.2g	0.8g		307 mg

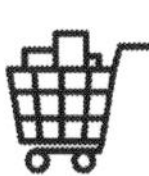

- 12 cups organic baby kale pre-washed
- 4 sliced boiled eggs
- 2 sliced cucumber
- 2 tbsp sesame seeds toasted

Healthy Spinach Salad Dressing

- 2 tbsp, of Dijon mustard
- ½ cup olive oil
- 1 tbsp. apple cider vinegar

1. Add kale, eggs, cucumber, and sesame seeds to a big salad dish.
2. Olive oil, , Dijon mustard, should all be combined in one little Mason jar. Shake until thoroughly blended while covering tightly.
3. Before serving, drizzle dressing over salad and gently toss. Sufficient for right away.

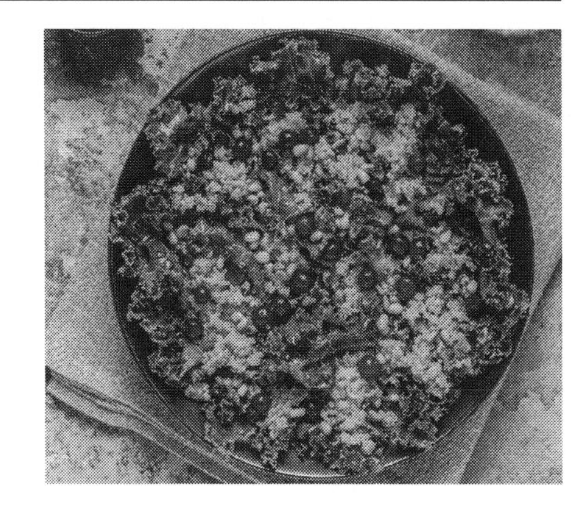

Storage:
Store the salad's components in the refrigerator, separated from the dressing, a maximum of two days. You can store dressing in a jar in the fridge for up to two weeks. Shake after warming up for ten minutes in a bowl of boiling water.

 8  15" 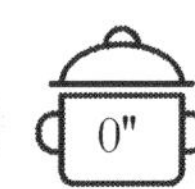 0"

4.2 Tomato Cucumber Lettuce Salad

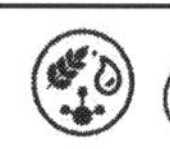 per serving 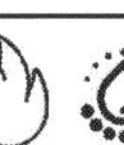 44 Cal 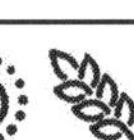 3.7g 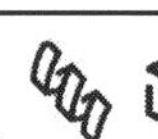 3.1g 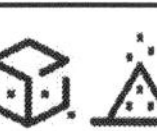 0.5g 1.4g 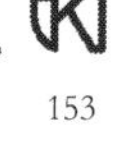 153 mg

- Cucumbers coarsely chopped – 2 medium
- Extra virgin olive oil, - 2 tbsp.
- Tomato roughly chopped – 1
- Salt – ½ tsp.
- Coarsely chopped lettuce, - 1 pound

1. Cucumber, tomato, lettuce, extra virgin olive oil, salt, should all be combined in a big bowl. The simplest method is to add ingredients both while you are preparing them, such as washing and chopping vegetables, and in the exact sequence that is mentioned.
2. Gently stir only enough to mix.
3. Immediately or within an hour, Serve it.

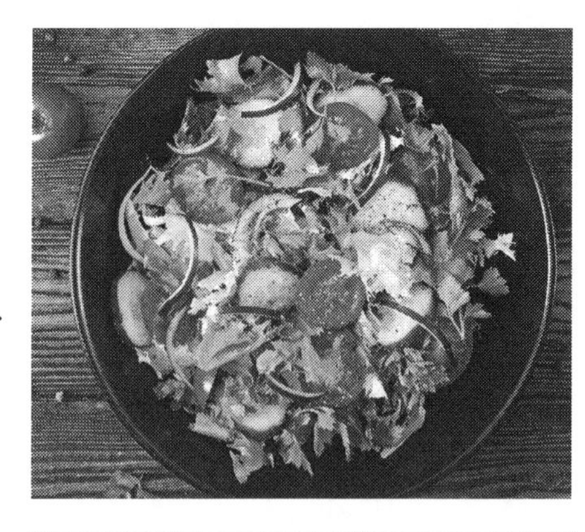

Storage:
Before serving, add oils, salt, and pepper to the dish of covered veggies that have been refrigerated..

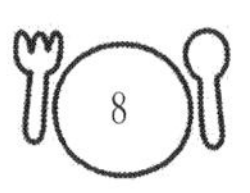 8 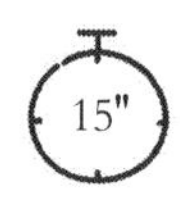 15" 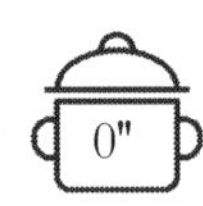 0"

4.3 Strawberry Kale Salad

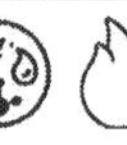 per serving 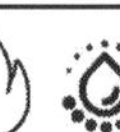 44 Cal 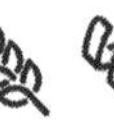 3.7g  3.1g 0.5g 1.4g 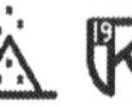 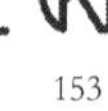 153 mg

- ½ lb strawberries hulled ,sliced in halves (quarters)
- 2 tbsp. feta cheese crumbled
- ¾ cups pecans
- 6 cups kale pre-washed

Dressing:

- Stevia – ¾ tbsp.
- Olive oil- 1 tbsp.
- Apple cider vinegar – 2 tbsp.

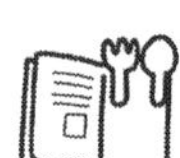

1. Pecans are added to a medium nonstick ceramic skillet that has been preheated. Toast, stirring regularly, for 3 minutes or until aromatic. To avoid burning nuts, quickly remove from heat.
2. Olive oil, stevia , apple cider vinegar, should all be combined in a small basin and whisked together. Place aside.
3. kale should be added to a big bowl along with the cheese, strawberries, and toasted pecans.
4. Dressing should be drizzled over the top, then gently mixed in. Serve it right away.

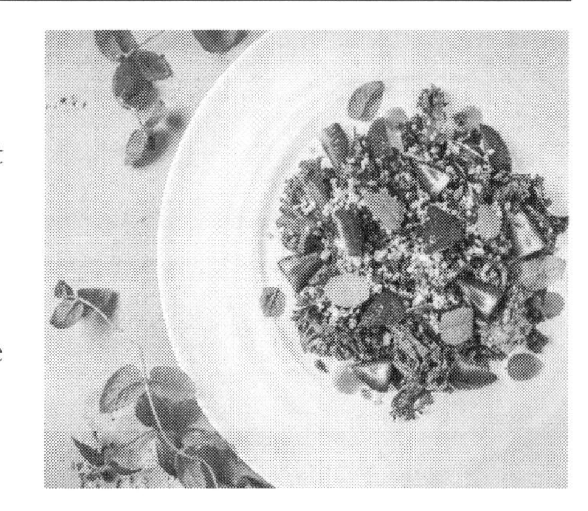

Storage:
This salad is best consumed within one to two hours of combining. Leftovers can be kept in the fridge for up to a day in an airtight container, although spinach will go mushy.

 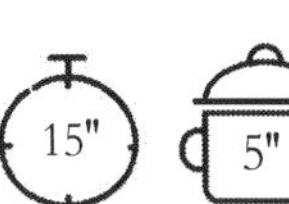

4.4 Lemon Kale Salad

 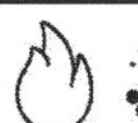 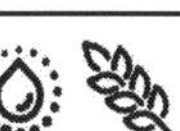 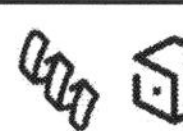 

per serving	144 Cal	12g	6.5g	4.1g	0.4g		305 mg

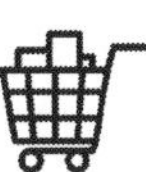

- Salt
- Walnut, coarsely chopped – ½ cup
- Kale chopped – 3 cups
- Lemon juice – 2 tbsp.
- Feta cheese -4 tbsp.
- Olive oil – 4 tbsp.

1. Remove the ribs from the kale, give it a cold water rinse, and then give it a salad spin.
2. Cut finely into stripes, then add to a sizable salad bowl.
3. Toast walnuts until fragrant on a medium heat in a skillet, stirring often. Include in a bowl of salad.
4. Toss toasted nuts and feta cheese into the salad dish.
5. Add olive oil, lemon juice, salt, to a small bowl. Use a fork to whisk, then pour over the salad.
6. Gently blend while stirring..

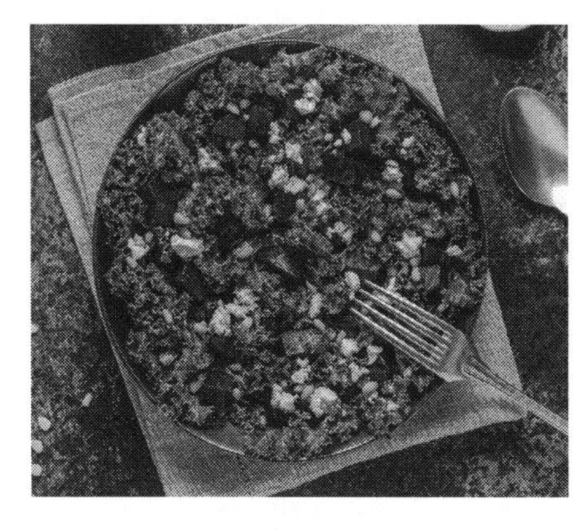

Storage:
Salad leftovers can be kept for up to 36 hours without getting mushy.

Make Ahead:
To make salad ahead, prepare the kale leaves and store them for up to 7 days in a zip-top bag.

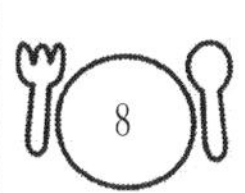  

4.5 Easy Arugula Salad

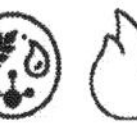 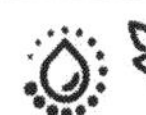 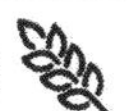 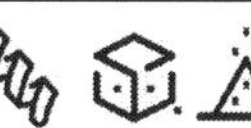 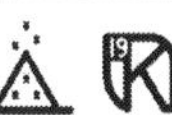 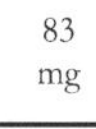

per serving	72 Cal	6.6g	1.3g	2.5g	1g		83 mg

- Arugula - 7-1/2 cups
- Lemon juice and zest -¾ tbsp,
- Salt- ¼ tsp.
- Olive oil – 1-1/2 tbsp.
- Feta cheese shavings - 12 tbsp.

1. Use a vegetable peeler to shave the feta cheese if required.
2. Arugula, olive oil, salt, optional lemon zest, and lemon juice should all be combined in a large basin. Toss everything with your hands so that it is all coated. feta shavings is next added, and everything is mixed by tossing briefly. If needed, salt to taste.

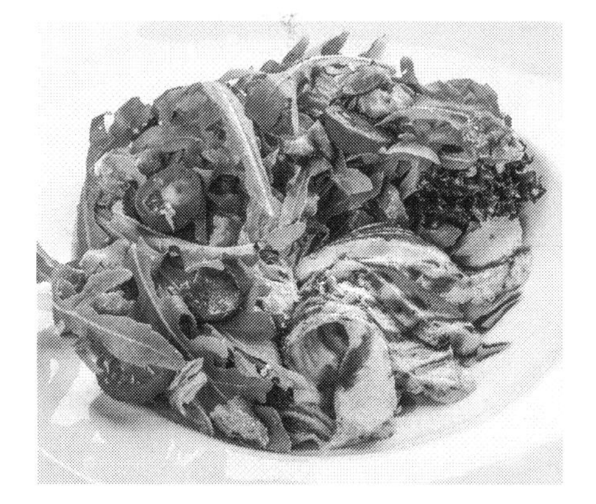

Storage:
Salad leftovers can be kept for up to 36 hours without getting mushy.

Make Ahead:
To make salad ahead, prepare the arugula leaves and store them for up to 7 days in a zip-top bag.

  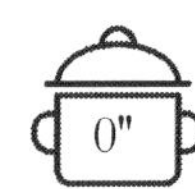

4.6 Simple Carrot Salad

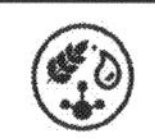 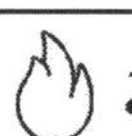 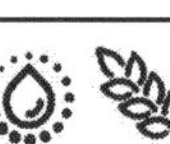 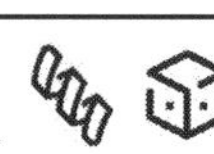 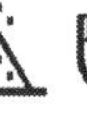 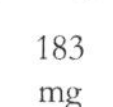

per serving	85 Cal	7.1g	5.6g	0.6g	2.7g	183 mg

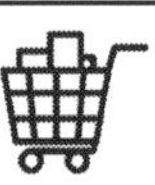

- Stevia – 1 tsp.
- Salt – ½ tsp.
- Apple cider vinegar – 1tbsp.
- Dijon mustard – ½ tbsp.
- Olive oil - 3 tbsp.
- Carrots, julienned - 3 cups
- Chopped cilantro -3 tbsp.

1. Apple cider vinegar, Dijon mustard, stevia, and salt should be combined in a basin. Mix in the olive oil gradually.
2. Peel the carrots and julienne them using a julienne peeler, a food processor's grating blade, or the box grater's large grate holes (this method works, but the pieces aren't as pretty).
3. Chop the cilantro finely.
4. Stirring the ingredients together, Fill the bowl with the dressing and all the vegetables..

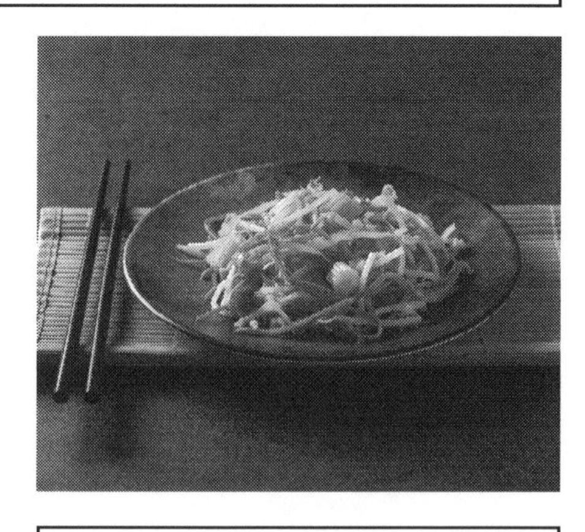

Storage:
Serve immediately or refrigerate for up to three days.

  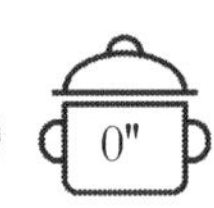

4.7 Broccoli Salad

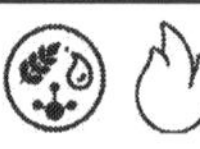 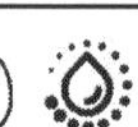 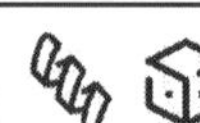 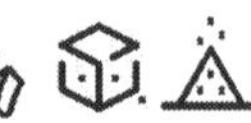 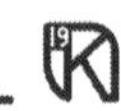

per serving	108 Cal	6.7g	10.4g	3.4g	2.7g	318 mg

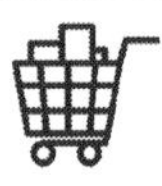

- 2.5 tbsp. apple cider vinegar
- ½ tbsp. sweetener like stevia
- ½ teaspoon salt
- ¼ cup sunflower seeds
- 2 carrot, julienned or grated
- 8 cups broccoli florets
- 8 tbsp of mayo
- 2 tsp. Dijon mustard

1. Reduce the broccoli to tiny florets.
2. Mayo, apple cider vinegar, stevia , Dijon mustard, and salt are all whisked together. Include with the vegetables and blend. To enable the flavors to mingle and the broccoli to soften, refrigerate for one hour (you can eat right away but the broccoli is crisp and has less of the traditional texture).
3. Add the sunflower seeds to the salad just before serving.

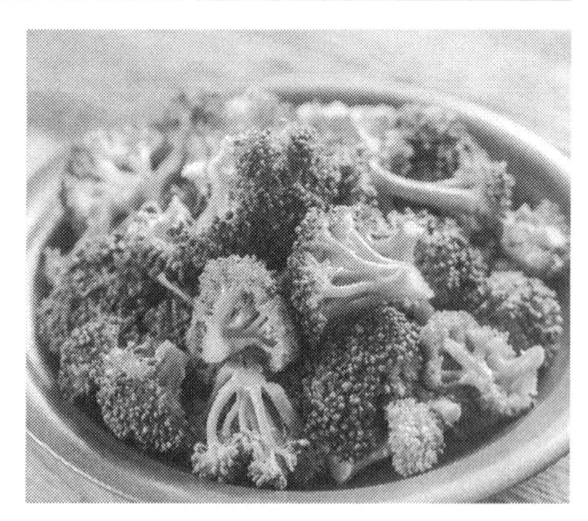

Storage:
Serve immediately or refrigerate for up to three days.

 4 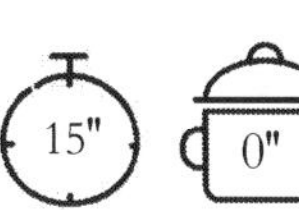 15"  0"

4.8 Sweet Potato Salad

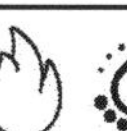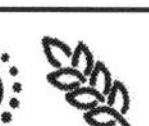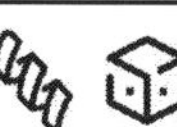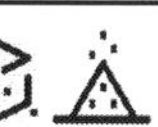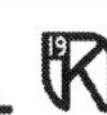

per serving	404 Cal	13.5g	66.6g	7.5g	2.4g		318 mg

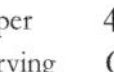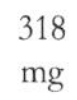

- 1 tsp. salt
- 1 cups baby arugula
- ¼ cup strawberries
- ¼ cup sunflower seed
- ¼ cup feta cheese crumbles
- 3/4 cups sweet potatoes
- 1 tbsp. olive oil

1. Before roasting the sweet potatoes, turn the oven on and heat it to 450 degrees.
2. When cutting the sweet potatoes into 3/4" cubes, keep the skin on. Sweet potatoes should be mixed with olive oil, and salt in a large basin.
3. Arrange the sweet potatoes in an even layer on a baking sheet that has been lined with parchment paper. The cubes should have roasted for around 25 minutes until they are fully cooked and have a browned bottom.
4. To assemble the salad, mix the baby arugula, strawberries, and roasted sweet potatoes in a bowl. Sunflower seeds and crumbled feta. Mix, and serve it

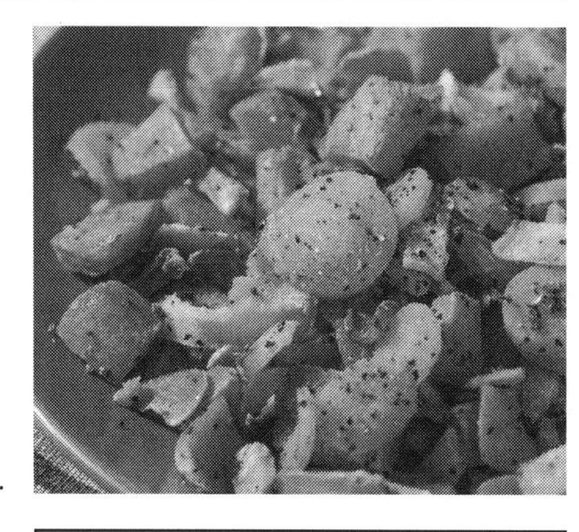

Storage:
Salad leftovers can be kept for up to 36 hours without getting mushy.

 4 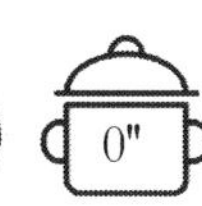 20" 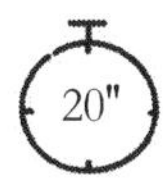 0"

4.9 Easy Vegetable Salad

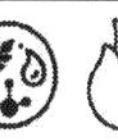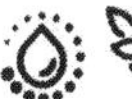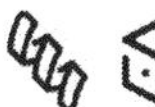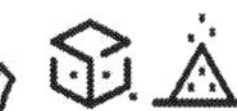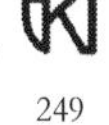

per serving	111 Cal	8.9g	6.6g	3.2g	2.8g		249 mg

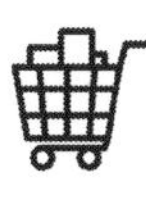

- 1 large bell pepper
- 1 tablespoon mustard
- 1 cup cucumber, diced
- 2 cups broccoli
- two teaspoons of oil
- two tbsp, of lemon juice
- and one teaspoon of salt

1. As said above, chop the vegetables, then add them to a big bowl. (Always keep the florets of the broccoli little.)
2. Toss with the salt, mustard, and oil, lemon juice., if desire add salt after tasting. Enjoy right away

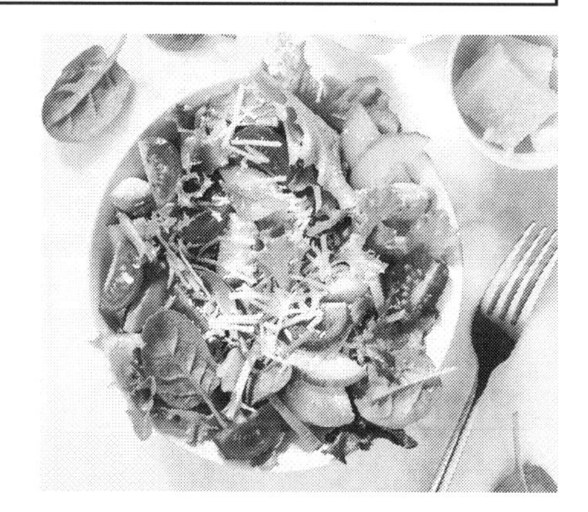

Storage:
For up to three days, keep in the refrigerator.

4.10 Broccoli Quinoa Salad

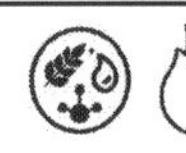 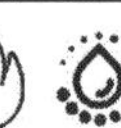 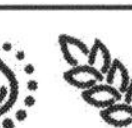 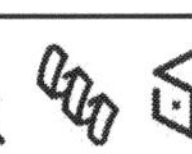 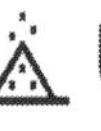

per serving	162 Cal	7.4g	20g	6.1g	1.8g	438 mg

- ¼ tsp salt + pinch
- Water – ¾ cup
- Olive oil – 3 tbsp.
- Quinoa uncooked – 1 cup
- Walnut chopped -1/2 cup
- Raw broccoli includes stems, cut into small pieces – ¾ lbs.
- Fresh, cilantro - ½ cup
- Lemon juice – ¼ tbsp.
- Zest of lemon – ¼

1. Mix the quinoa, water, and a dash of salt in a medium pot. Cook for ten minutes with a cover on after comminute to a boil and reducing the heat. removing the heat after 5 minutes of standing and fluff with a fork. Set aside.
2. Meanwhile, add walnut to a small skillet that has been preheated over low heat. Toast with periodic stirring until golden brown. Place aside.
3. Broccoli should be added to a food processor and cut fully in batches.
4. Add the cooked quinoa, toasted walnuts, cilantro, salt , olive oil, juice and zest of lemon, into a big bowl.
5. Gently mix everything together, and if you have time, let the salad cool in the refrigerator for about an hour. Serve chilled.

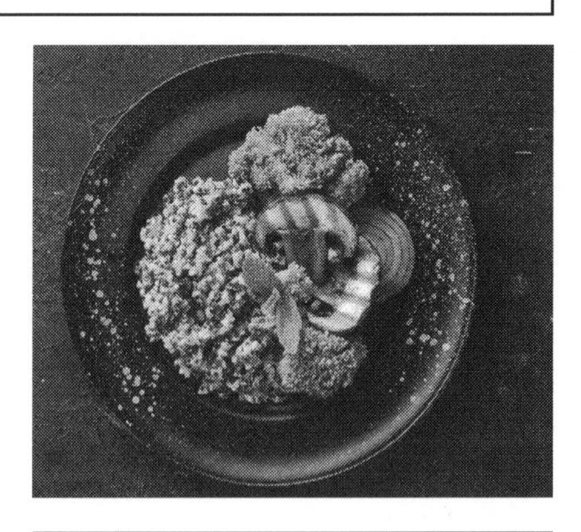

Storage:
For up to three days, keep in the refrigerator.

4.11 Chicken Salad

 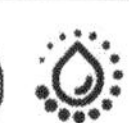 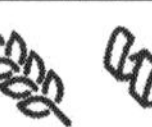 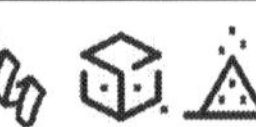 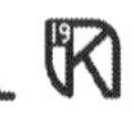

per serving	100 Cal	3.9g	1.7g	13.8g	0.5g	118 mg

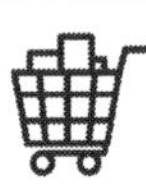

- Lemon juice - 1 tsp
- Salt
- Parsley – 6 tablespoon
- Walnuts – ½ cup
- Chicken -¾ cups
- Mayo -1/4 cup
- Mustard- 1 tsp

1. Walnuts should be put to a small skillet and toasted until aromatic and browned over low to medium heat, flipping often. After being moved to a chopping board and given some time to cool, chop thinly.
2. In a medium bowl, mix the chicken, parsley, mayo, mustard, lemon juice, and salt with the toasted walnuts. Mix well, taste, and make any required salt adjustments.
3. Salad tastes best when it is cold, so refrigerate for at least two hours.
4. Serve the chicken salad on with greens or quinoa.

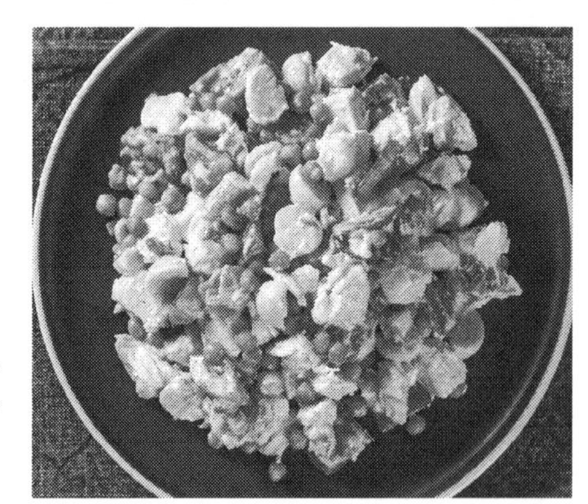

Storage:
You can keep food in the refrigerator for up to five days if it's sealed tightly.

 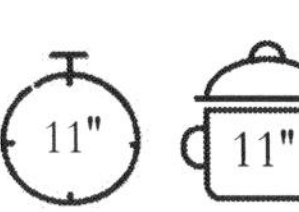

4.12 Egg Salad

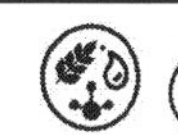 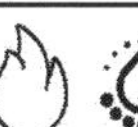 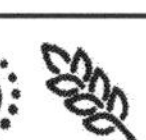 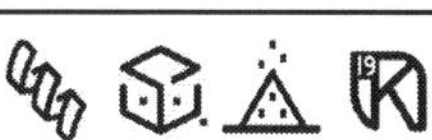 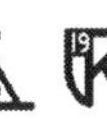

per serving | 176 Cal | 12.2g | 2.7g | 12.8g | 1.5g | 155 mg

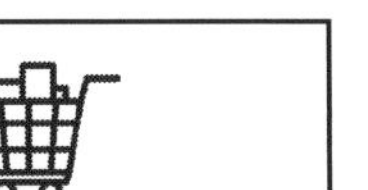

- 1-1/2 tablespoon mayo
- ½ tablespoon mustard
- 1 tablespoon parsley
- Pinch of salt
- 7 eggs cooked

1. Peel the eggs after cooling. Add them to a medium bowl after chopping them roughly or finely as you choose.
2. Salt, mustard, parsley, , and mayo can all be added.
3. Combine by using a spoon to stir slowly.
4. Serve the egg salad right away, though it tastes best after chilling for an hour

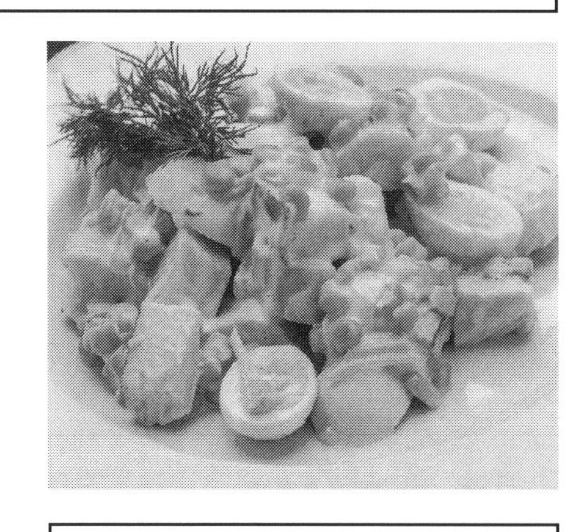

Storage:
You can keep food in the refrigerator for up to five days if it's sealed tightly

4.13 Smoked Salmon

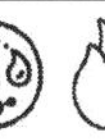 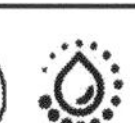 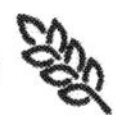 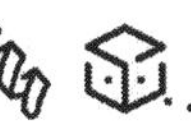 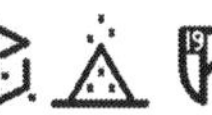 

per serving | 283 Cal | 19.9g | 8.7g | 18.4g | 0.3g | 529 mg

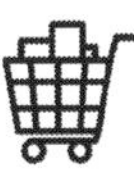

- Sesame seeds preferably toasted - 1 tbsp
- Big handful salad greens, arugula or kale
- Lemon juice - 1 tbsp
- Smoked salmon preferably wild – 3 slices
- Cucumber sliced – ¼
- Olive oil – 1 tbsp.

1. Add salmon and greens to a medium bowl. Salmon can be further stretched if it is sliced or torn into little pieces.
2. Add cucumber.
3. Olive oil and lemon juice are drizzled on top along with sesame seeds. Be blown away by a gentle toss!

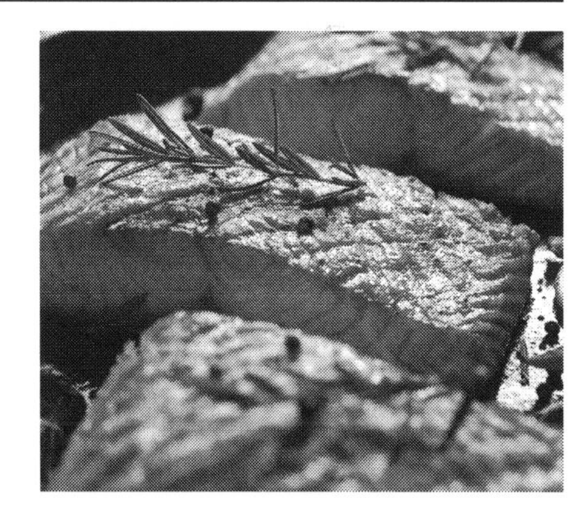

Storage:
You can keep food in the refrigerator for up to five days if it's sealed tightly

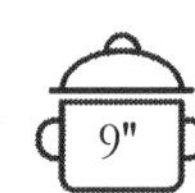

4.14 Healthy Cucumber Salad

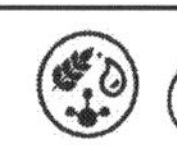 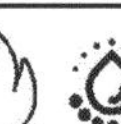 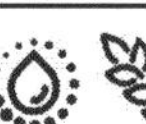 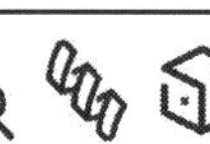 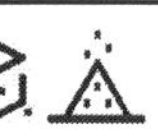 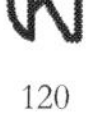

per serving | 42 Cal | 3.6g | 2.8g | 0.5g | 1.3g | 120 mg

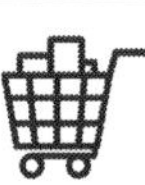

- 2 English cucumbers sliced
- ¼ cup cilantro chopped
- 1 tablespoon oil
- ½ tablespoon vinegar
- ¼ tsp salt

1. In a large bowl, combine the cucumbers, cilantro, olive oil, vinegar, salt.
2. Stir everything together completely. This salad is best enjoyed right away because the cucumber tends to become watery with age. But you can combine everything (salt not included) and refrigerate for up to 24 hours. Stir in seasoning just before serving.

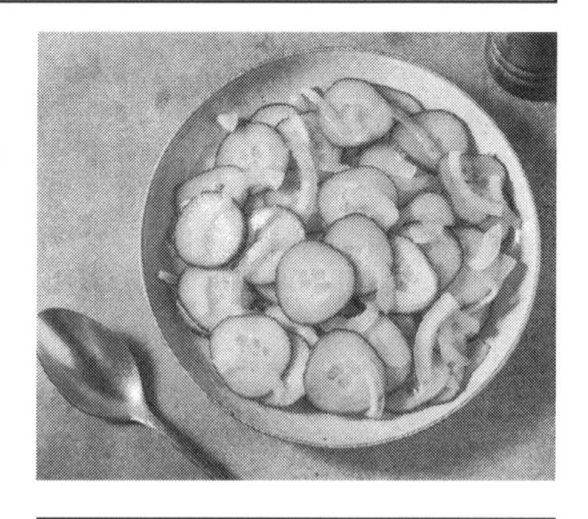

Storage:
You can keep food in the refrigerator for up to five days if it's sealed tightly

4.15 Zesty Quinoa Salad

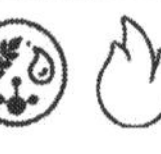 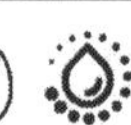 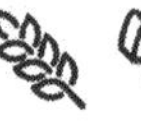 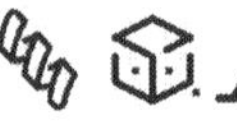 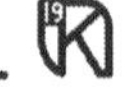 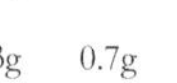 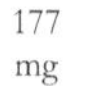

per serving | 142 Cal | 7.6g | 16g | 3.3g | 0.7g | 177 mg

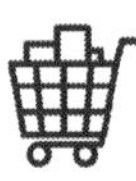

- 3/4 cup water
- 1.5 tbsp, olive oil
- ½ lemon, juiced
- ½ tsp. salt
- 1 medium tomato
- 4 tbsp of chopped fresh cilantro
- ½ cup quinoa

1. Bring water and quinoa to a boil in a saucepan. After quinoa is cooked and water is absorbed, lower heat to medium-low, cover, and simmer for 10 to 15 minutes. sufficient for cooling.
2. Olive oil, lime juice, salt, should all be combined in a small bowl as you wait.
3. In a sizable bowl, mix the quinoa, tomatoes. Toss the quinoa mixture with the dressing to coat. Add the cilantro and season with salt. Serve for right away or let the food cool in the fridge.

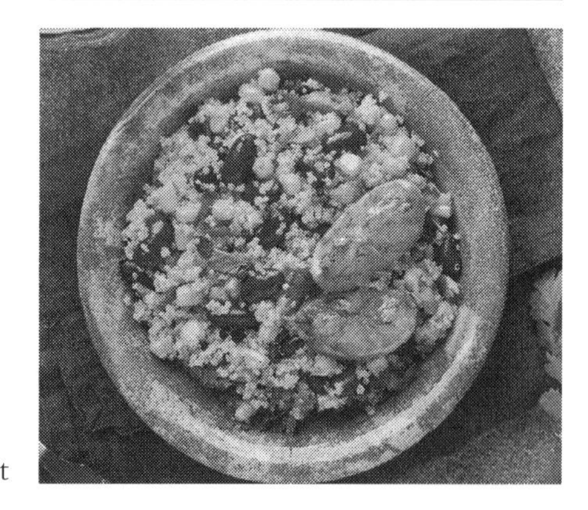

Storage:
You can keep food in the refrigerator for up to five days if it's sealed tightly.

CHAPTER 5

VEGETARIAN DISHES

5.1 Bamboo Shoot Stir Fry Recipe

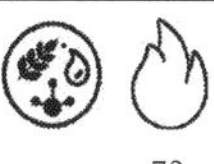 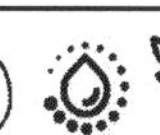 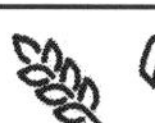 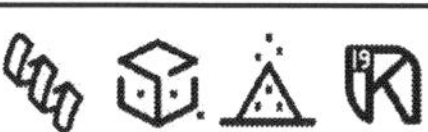 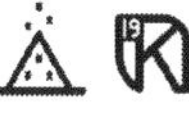

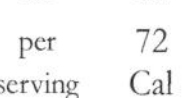 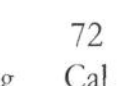 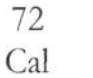 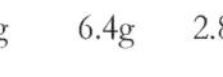 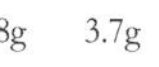 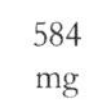

per serving	72 Cal	5g	6.4g	2.8g	3.7g		584 mg

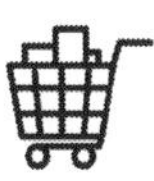

- 8 cups Bamboo shoots , julienned
- 2 cups Bell Peppers
- 4 tbsp. Olive Oil
- Salt

1. To start cooking bamboo shoots, heat a skillet should be heated to medium.
2. After the olive oil warms up
3. Add cook the bamboo shoots for 2 minutes.
4. Add the salt-required bell peppers, and sauté until all the veggies are tender but still crisp.
5. After tasting for salt, Serve for the recipe for bamboo shoot stir-fry with quinoa.

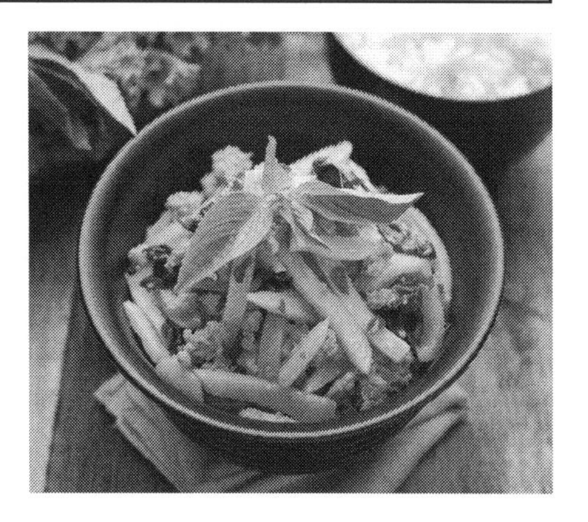

Storage:
For around two months, stir fry can be frozen.

Reheat:
Stir-fry can be safely heated. Just remember to keep any leftover stir-fries in the refrigerator or freezer until you're ready to reheat them, as stir-fries left out at room temperature are probably not safe to eat.

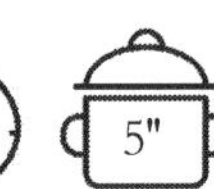

5.2 Bean Sprout Stir Fry

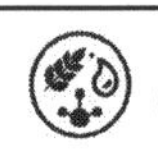 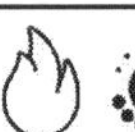 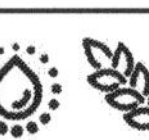 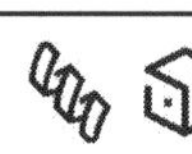 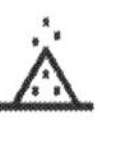 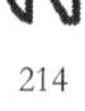

per serving	53 Cal	2.9g	4.7g	4.8g	0g	214 mg

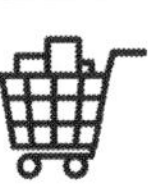

- 1 tsp oil to cook
- ½ pound bean sprouts, hair removed
- Salt to taste

1. Add oil when its heat . Add the bean sprouts right away and stir-fry them, swiftly turning them over. Verify the seasoning. Serve right away.

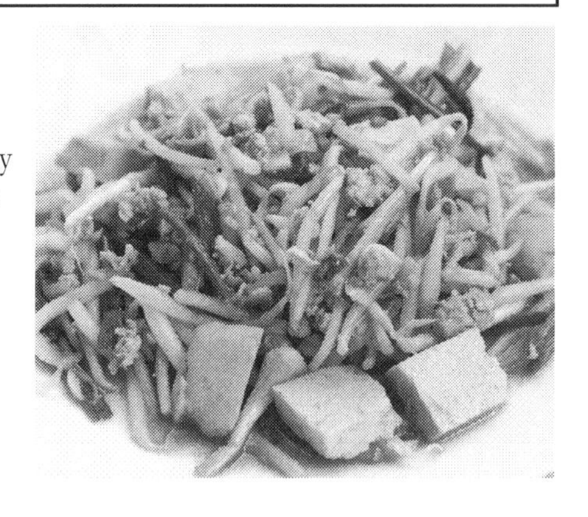

Storage:
For around two months, stir fry can be frozen.

Reheat:
Stir-fry can be safely heated. Just remember to keep any stir-fries left out at room temperature are probably not safe to consume, so store any leftovers in the freezer or refrigerator until you're ready to reheat them.

5.3 Roasted Lemon Broccoli

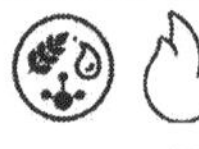 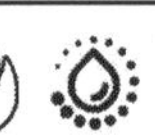 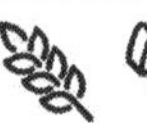 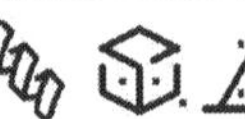  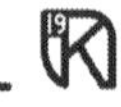

per serving	57 Cal	4.7g	3.1g	1.3g	0.8g	145 mg

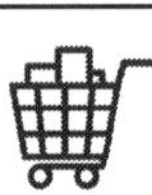

- 1 head broccoli, separated into florets
- 1 teaspoon garlic infused oil
- ½ teaspoon sea salt
- ¼ teaspoon lemon juice

1. The oven should be set to 400 degrees Fahrenheit.
2. Combine the broccoli florets with the garlic-infused oil and sea salt in a large bowl. On a baking sheet, arrange the broccoli in a single layer.
3. Bake the florets in the preheated oven for 15 to 20 minutes, or until they are tender enough to puncture with a fork. After removal, transfer to a serving dish.
4. To give broccoli a cool, tangy flavor, liberally sprinkle lemon juice over it just before serving.

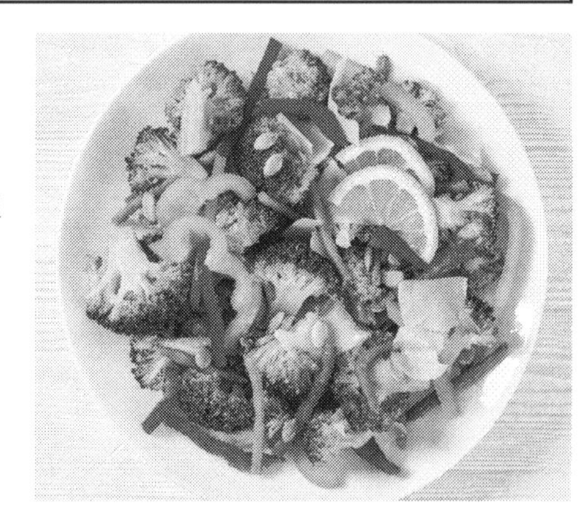

Storage:
Storing roasted broccoli in the refrigerator for no more than a day or two.

Reheat:
Although it is a possibility, microwave reheating of roasted broccoli does not produce the greatest texture.

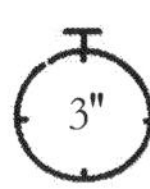

5.4 Lemon Sauteed Cabbage

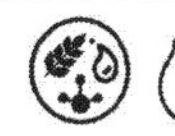
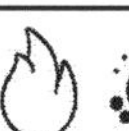
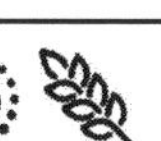
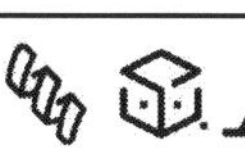

per serving | 67 Cal | 4.7g | 6.8g | 1.2g | 3g | 159 mg

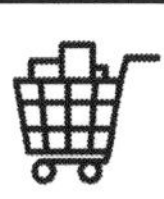

- 3 cups cabbage, core removed and shredded
- 2 tablespoons garlic infused oil
- 1 tsp salt
- Half a lemon,

1. Warm the oil in a large skillet or Dutch oven over medium-high heat. Add salt and cabbage. Even though there may first seem to be too much cabbage in the pan, it will wilt as it cooks.
2. Cook for 10 to 15 minutes, stirring periodically, until the cabbage is soft and part of it starts to become light brown.
3. Add lemon slices should be used to squeeze juice over the cabbage. When necessary, add extra salt, and lemon juice after tasting.

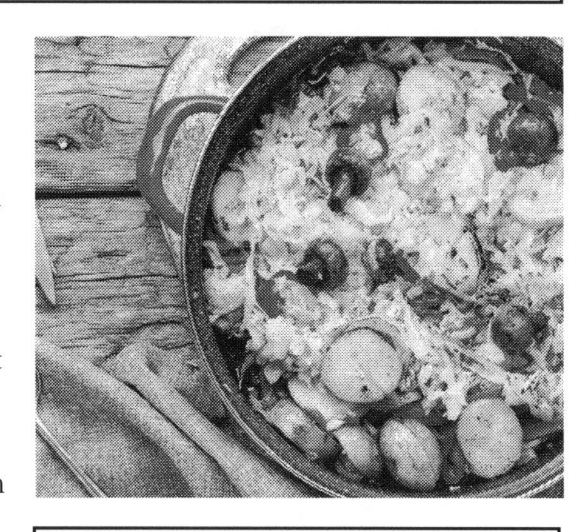

Storage:
Sautéed cabbage can be kept in the refrigerator for If maintained in an airtight container, it can last for up to a week.

Reheat:
A microwave-safe bowl or plate can be used to reheat sautéed cabbage. Just heat it up until it's warm.

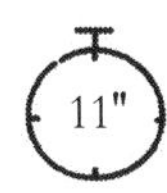

5.5 Homemade Coleslaw

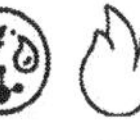

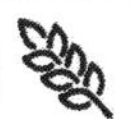
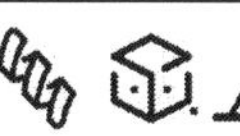
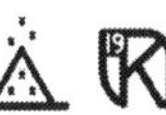

per serving | 124 Cal | 9.9g | 9g | 0.5g | 3g | 65 mg

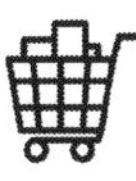

- ¾ cup mayo
- ¼ cup vinegar
- 4 teaspoons Dijon mustard
- 1.5 tablespoon stevia
- Kosher salt
- ½ head green cabbage, thinly sliced
- 1 large carrots, grated

1. Mayo, vinegar, Dijon mustard, stevia, should be combined in a whisk. To taste, add salt to the food. Mix in cabbage ,carrots into a bowl and add dressing on them.
2. Until ready to serve, refrigerate after wrapping in plastic wrap.

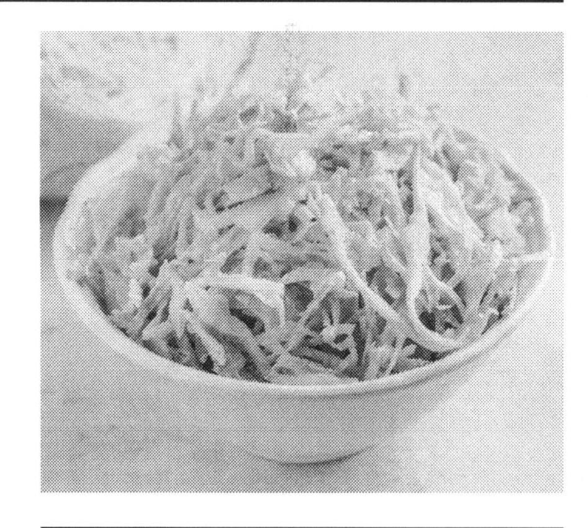

Storage:
Coleslaw can be kept in the refrigerator for If maintained in an airtight container, it can last for up to a week.

Reheat:
A microwave-safe bowl or plate can be used to reheat sautéed cabbage. Just heat it up until it's warm.

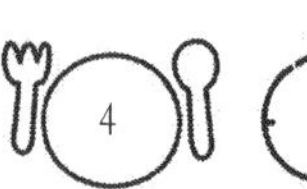

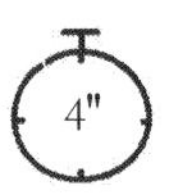

5.6 Sautéed Eggplant

 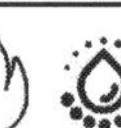 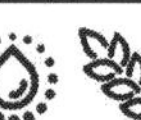 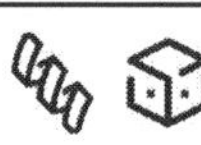 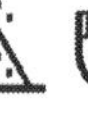 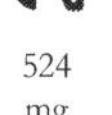

per serving | 78 Cal | 2.7g | 13.5g | 2.2g | 6.9g | 524 mg

- 1 Eggplant
- ¼ tsp Garlic infused oil
- 1/4 tsp Sea salt

1. Cut circles out of the eggplant that are about 1/4 inch (6 mm) thick. Only remove the leafy end once you have finished slicing so that you have more to hold onto. Pat the slices dry if they are wet.
2. Garlic Garlic infused oil, sea salt, should be liberally sprinkled on both sides of the slices of eggplant.
3. A 12-inch skillet with two teaspoons of olive oil heated over low to medium heat. Add the eggplant slices in a single layer while working in batches. Cook eggplant for 3-6 minutes on each side, or until it is tender, browned, and caramelized. Follow the same procedure, adding 1-2 teaspoons of oil every batch, with the remaining eggplant pieces.

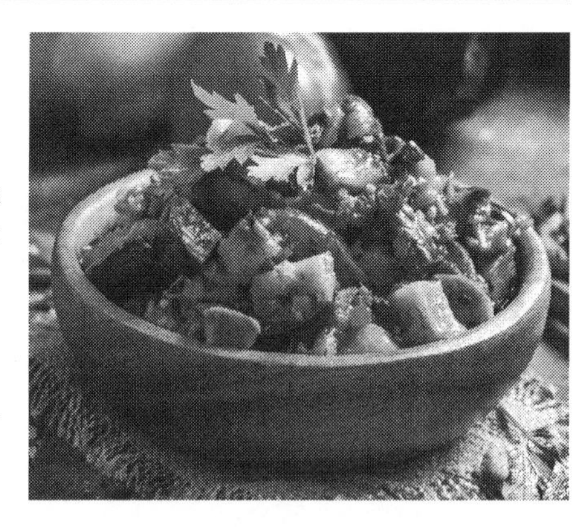

Storage:
Sautéed Eggplant can be kept in the refrigerator for If maintained in an airtight container, it can last for up to a week.

Reheat:
A microwave-safe bowl or plate can be used to reheat sautéed eggplant. Just heat it up until it's warm.

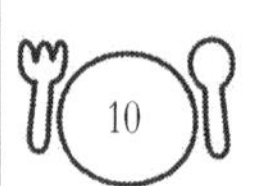

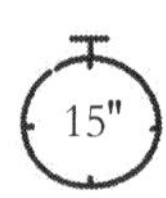

5.7 Simple Skillet Green Beans

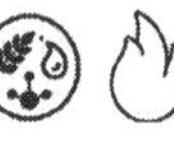 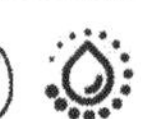 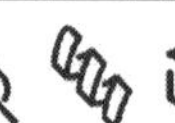 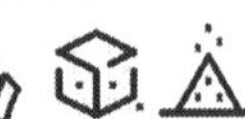 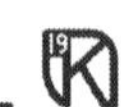

per serving | 92 Cal | 5.8g | 10.1g | 2.6g | 1.9g | 289 mg

- 4 tbsp oil
- 3 lbs of trimmed green beans
- 3/4 teaspoon salt
- 3.5 tbsp of water

1. Place a large skillet over medium-high heat and heat the oil.
2. Green beans should start to blister and turn brown after 5 to 7 minutes of cooking. Continue cooking while tossing often.
3. Add salt and stir continuously for about 30 seconds, or until it is fragrant and starting to brown. After adding water, immediately cover. The beans should be brilliant green and crisp-tender after they are finished cooking for 1 to 2 minutes under cover. Serve immediately.

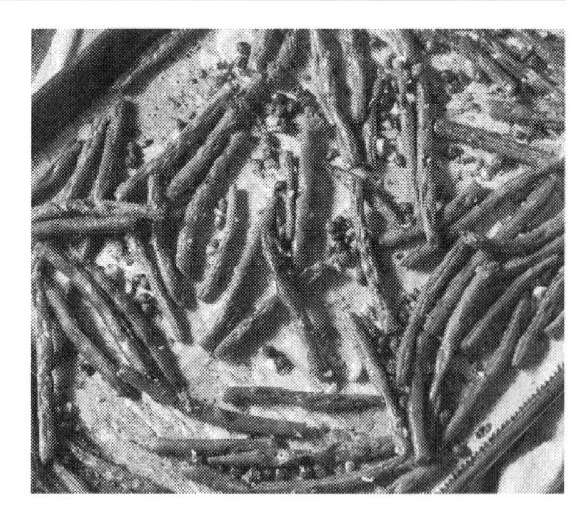

Storage:
Cooked green beans can be kept in the fridge for 3 to 5 days when kept properly..

Reheat:
If you've already cooked the green beans, reheat them as soon as you're ready to Sufficient for, using the least amount of cooking time as you can.

 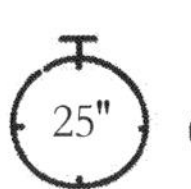 

5.8 Potato and Green Bean

 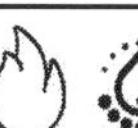  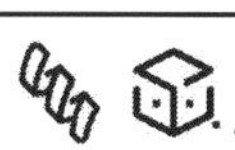 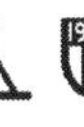

per serving	102 Cal	2.6g	18.2g	2.4g	1.1g	489 mg

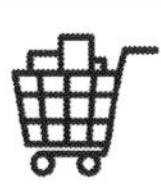

- kosher salt
- Green beans -¼ lb.
- small new potatoes -2 1/2 lb.
- mustard -2 tbsp.
- vinegar -¼ cup
- cilantro -¼ cup
- oil – 2 tbsp

1. Add beans after bringing a big saucepan of water to a boil. Cook for about 2-3 minutes, or until the greens are bright and crisp but still soft. To stop the cooking of cooked beans, immediately submerge them in a bowl of ice water. After fully cooling, rinse the beans in a colander.
2. In a sizable Ziploc bag, combine the diced potatoes, oil, mustard, vinegar, and cilantro . To coat, shake. Potatoes are added to a heated skillet over medium-high heat. Cook, stirring periodically, until the food begins to brown. Reduce heat to medium-low to avoid overbrowning potatoes before they are cooked through. sometimes stir. Cook till soft and golden. Add salt, taste along with the well-drained green beans. Cook for a further 3 to 5 minutes.

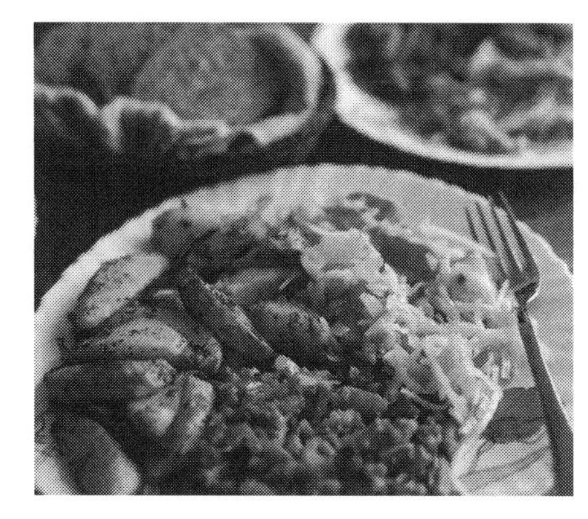

Storage:
Cooked green beans and potato can be kept in the fridge for 3 to 5 days when kept properly.

Reheat:
If you've already cooked the green beans, reheat them as soon as you're ready to Sufficient for, using the least amount of cooking time as you can.

 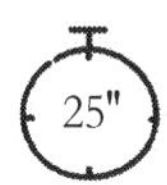 

5.9 Green Beans with Orange and Walnut Gremolata

 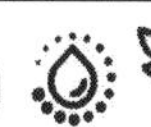 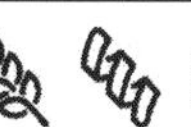 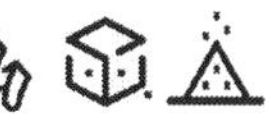

per serving	115 Cal	8.3g	9.2g	4.1g	1.7g	300 mg

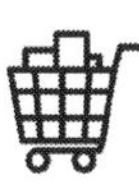

- 1 lb. green beans
- 2 tbsp oil
- 2 teaspoons cilantro
- ¼ cup roasted walnuts, roughly chopped
- 1 teaspoon orange zest
- 6 tablespoon parsley

1. Bring water in a big pot to a boil. Large basin filled with ice water. Green beans should be cooked in batches for 3 to 4 minutes until just tender after adding 1 tablespoon salt to boiling water. After draining and setting aside, add green beans to the cold water to cool.
2. Oil, cilantro should be heated for one minutes over medium heat in a small skillet. Add the orange zest, walnuts, and parsley after the mixture has been removed off the heat.
3. Provide warm or room temperature green beans.

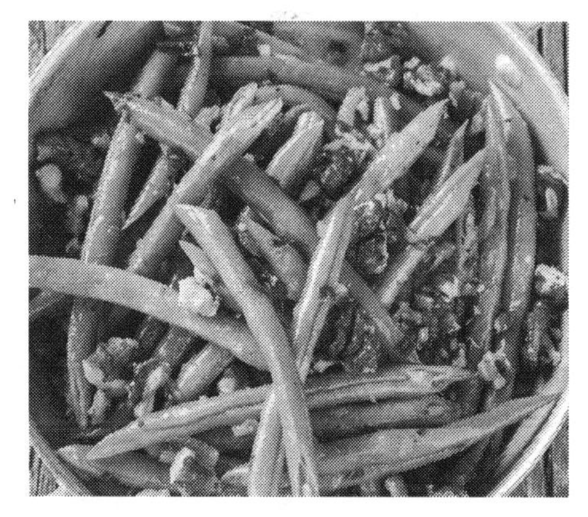

Storage:
Green Beans with Orange and Walnut Gremolatacan be kept in the fridge for 3 to 5 days when kept properly.

Reheat:
If you've already cooked the green beans, reheat them as soon as you're ready to Sufficient for, using the least amount of cooking time as you can.

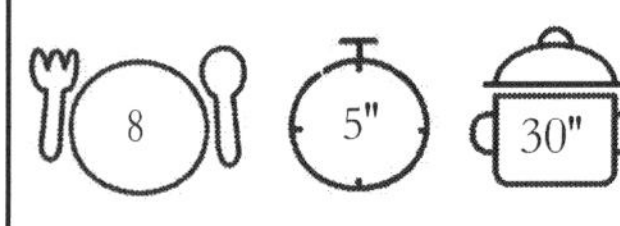 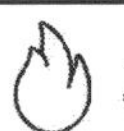 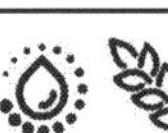 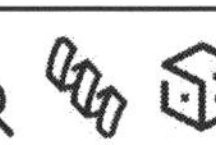 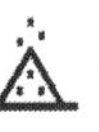

5.10 Curried Pumpkin

8 | 5" | 30"

per serving | 147 Cal | 5.4g | 24.2g | 3.2g | 3.2g | 668 mg

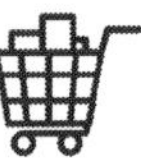

- Oil - 2 tbsp.
- fresh cilantro
- Curry powder - 2tsp.
- Salt - 1 tsp.
- Pumpkin - 2 lbs.
- Red potato - 1
- Water - ¾ cup

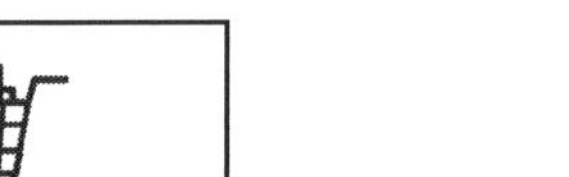

1. In a big pan, heat the oil over medium-high heat. Curry powder and salt are optional. It is advised to cook the potatoes and pumpkin for five minutes while stirring constantly.
2. After incorporating the water, lower the heat to medium. Replace the lid and cook the potatoes and pumpkin for a further 5 to 10 minutes, or until they are tender.
3. Cilantro makes a fantastic garnish.

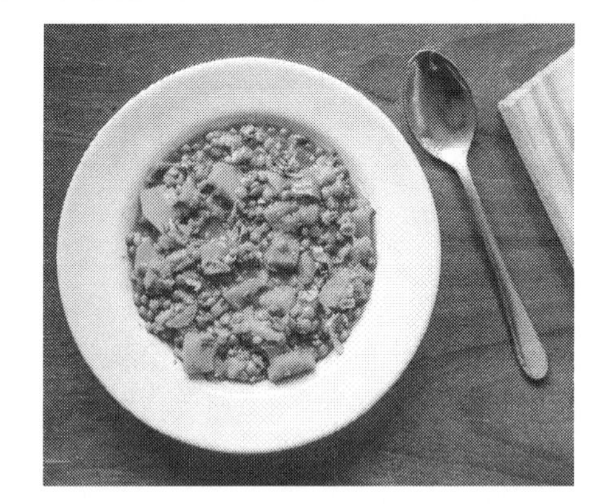

Storage:
Pumpkin can be frozen for up to three months, whether it is raw or cooked. Pumpkin should be diced and kept in freezer bags or containers.

Reheat:
You'll need a microwave, an oven, or a burner to reheat takeout curry. Put your curry onto a microwave-safe dish and heat for around 5 minutes if you're using one..

 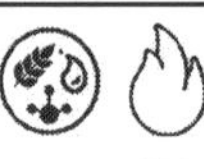 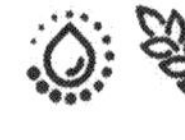 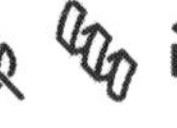 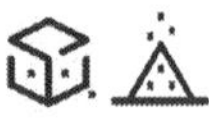 

5.11 Baked Pumpkin with Olive Oil

2 | 18" | 28"

per serving | 100 Cal | 4.8g | 14.2g | 2.3g | 3.1g | 765 mg

- 1.5 lbs. whole pumpkin
- 0.5 tbsp, garlic infused oil
- ½ teaspoon salt

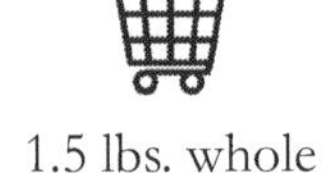

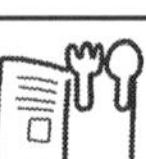

1. Set the oven temperature to 425 degrees. Oven rack should be placed in the bottom position. A large baking sheet with a rim can be lined with parchment paper.
2. Pumpkin cleanup and drying. Put it in the microwave and heat on high for one minutes to soften.
3. Carefully split the pumpkin in half using a chef's knife that is extremely sharp and back-and-forth sawing motions.
4. Make use of a large metal spoon to scoop out the pulp and seeds. If any stubborn chunks of pulp remain, cut them with kitchen scissors. If you wish to make roasted pumpkin seeds, save the seeds.
5. Discard the ends and use the sharp knife to cut each pumpkin half into four moon-shaped slices that are each one inch thick.
6. Peel the skin from each slice of pumpkin using a vegetable peeler, and then chop each slice into chunks of one inch.
7. Put the pumpkin chunks in a big bowl. After pouring the garlic infused oil and salt, evenly distribute them over the pumpkin chunks by using a large spoon or your hands.
8. Place the prepared baking sheet with the pumpkin cubes in a thin layer.. They should be tender after baking for around 30 minutes, stirring them halfway through. Serve immediately.

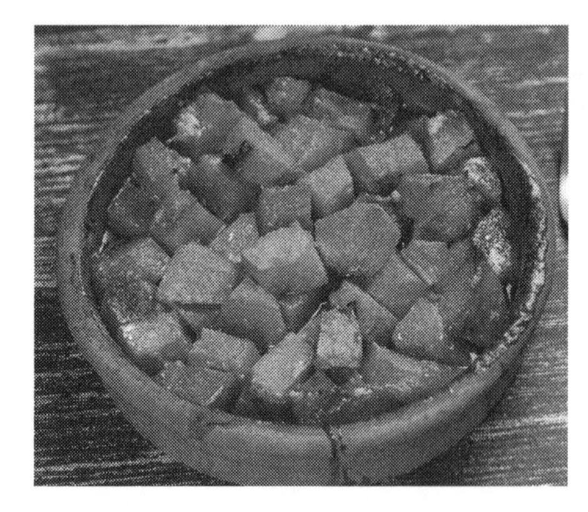

Storage:
Put frozen zucchini pieces in a sizable gallon-sized ziplock bag, and keep in the freezer for up to 3–4 months.

Reheat:
Reheat until well warmed through over low heat in a skillet on the stove top, at 350 degrees Fahrenheit in the oven, or in the microwave.

2

11"

11"

5.12 Sautéed Zucchini

 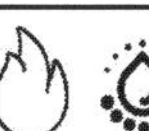 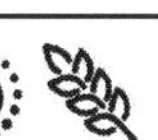 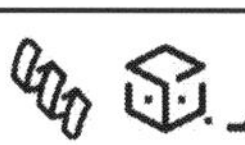 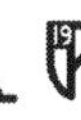

per serving | 147 Cal | 5.4g | 24.2g | 3.2g | 3.2g | 668 mg

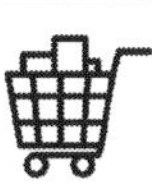

- 0.5 tbsp. oil
- 3 zucchini,
- 1 teaspoon oregano, dried
- salt
- 1/8 cup grated feta cheese

1. Heat the oil in a big skillet on a medium heat.
2. Add oregano and zucchini. The zucchini should be cooked for around 10 minutes, or until it is soft. To season the food, add salt.
3. Enough for a hot meal with feta cheese on top.

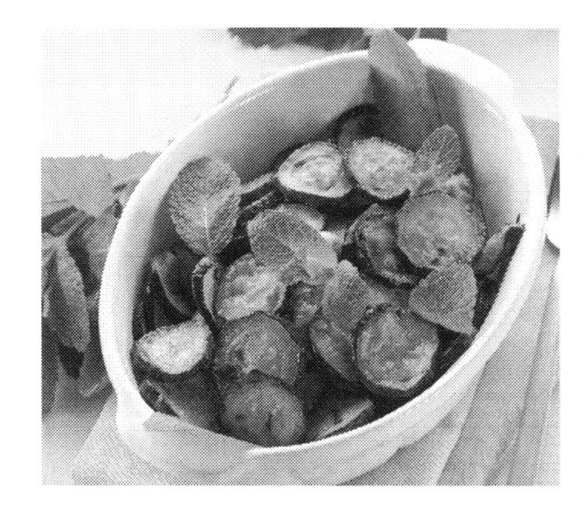

Storage:
Put frozen zucchini pieces in a sizable gallon-sized ziplock bag, and keep in the freezer for up to 3–4 months.

Reheat:
You'll need a microwave, an oven, or a burner to reheat takeout curry. Put your curry onto a microwave-safe dish and heat for around 5 minutes if you're using one..

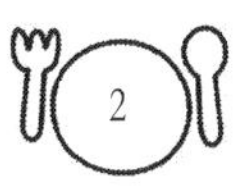
2

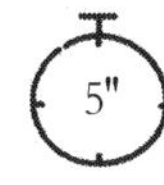
5"

10"

5.13 Sautéed Yellow Squash

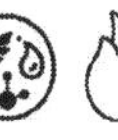 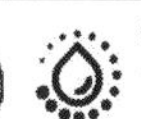 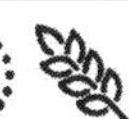 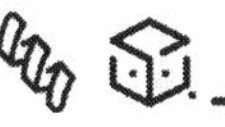 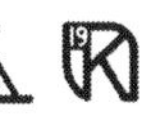

per serving | 77 Cal | 7.2g | 3.5g | 1.3g | 1.8g | 276 mg

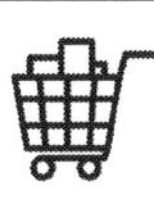

- Cilantro - 1/4 cup
- Fresh basil leaves,- 5
- Lemon juice – ½ tbsp
- Yellow squash sliced into 1/2-inch slices, - 1 medium
- Olive oil - 1 tbsp.
- Sea salt – ½ tsp.

1. Heat a large skillet over medium-high. Use olive oil.
2. After the oil has hot, add the yellow squash. Squash is stirred. For five minutes, cook. After flipping the squash over, heat for an additional 4 minutes while stirring constantly.
3. The pan needs to be filled with cilantro. After blending, cook for a further two minutes.
4. After removing the squash from the heat, stir in the basil, lemon juice, and sea salt. Stir and enough for immediately.

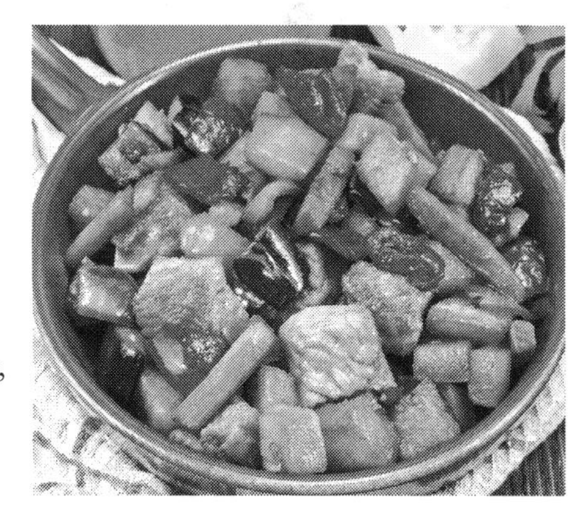

Storage:
Put frozen squash pieces in a sizable gallon-sized ziplock bag, and keep in the freezer for up to 3–4 months.

Reheat:
Reheat until well warmed through over low heat in a skillet on the stove top, at 350 degrees Fahrenheit

 3  11"  11"

5.14 Grilled Vegetables

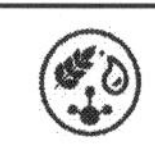 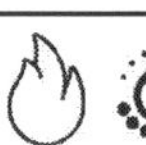 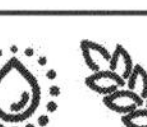 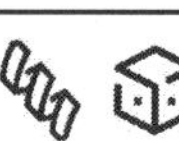 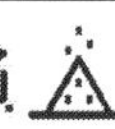 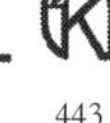

per serving	162 Cal	14.5g	9.1g	2.2g	5.2g		443 mg

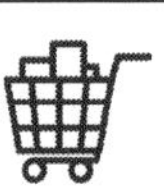

- Zucchini, - 2
- Yellow squash -2
- Bell peppers - 2
- Oil – 2 tbsp.
- Lemon juice - 2 tbsp.
- Dried basil - 1 tbsp.
- Optional: cilantro, thinly sliced - 1 tbsp.

1. Set the grill or grill pan's heat to medium-high.
2. In a sizable mixing basin, combine the zucchini, squash, and bell pepper along with the olive oil, salt, cilantro.
3. Vegetables should be threaded onto skewers.
4. They should be cook for 3 to 5 minutes, or until grill lines appear, on the grill. To get them blackened, Cook them for an additional 3 to 5 minutes after flipping them.. Place on a sizable platter or cutting board right away after being removed. Give vegetables a minutes or two to cool.
5. Take the skewers of vegetables out of the oven. Lemon juice should be drizzled on top. Add optional cilantro on top, if desired.
6. Serve it right away.

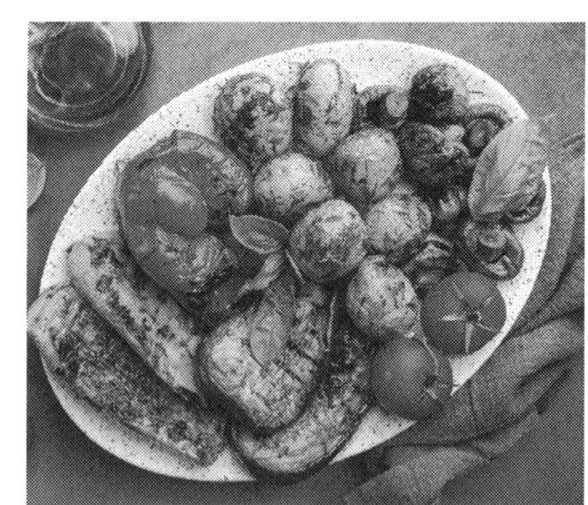

Storage:
Put frozen squash pieces in a sizable gallon-sized ziplock bag, and keep in the freezer for up to 3–4 months.

Reheat:
Layer them in shallow pans and place in the fridge. Plastic wrap each layer, then store for up to two days.

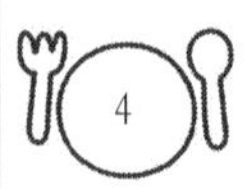 4 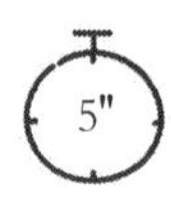 5" 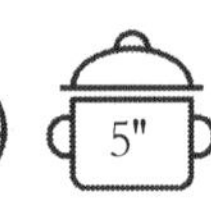 5"

5.15 Skillet Kale with Lemon

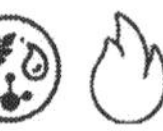 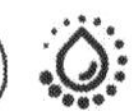 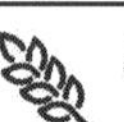 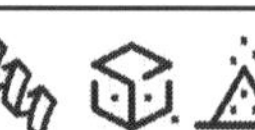 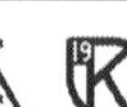 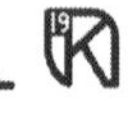

per serving	85 Cal	7.1g	6.2g	1.3g	0.7g		205 mg

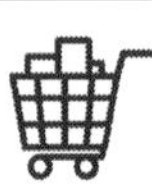

- 1 bunches kale, any variety
- 1 tbsp, olive oil
- ¼ teaspoon salt
- Juice of 1 small lemon

1. Kale leaves can be separated from their stems by using your hands. Chop the leaves roughly. Do not dry them after rinsing.
2. In a sizable, wide, high-sided sauté pan, heat the oil until shimmering. Stirring constantly, Until all kale is added should be done a few handfuls each time, stirring to help it wither after each addition.
3. Add the salt and stir-fry. 5 minutes, with the lid closed, simmer the kale, stirring regularly, until it is barely soft. Serve for after stirring in the lemon juice and turning off the heat.

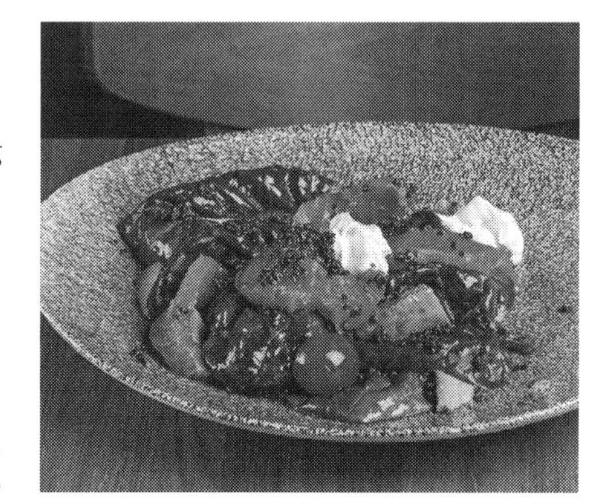

Storage:
up to five days when kept chilled in an airtight container.

Reheat:
Layer them in shallow pans and place in the fridge. Plastic wrap each layer, then store for up to two days.

CHAPTER 6

SOUP RECIPES

6.1 Roasted Squash Soup

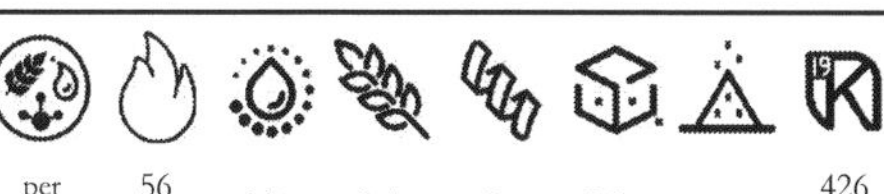
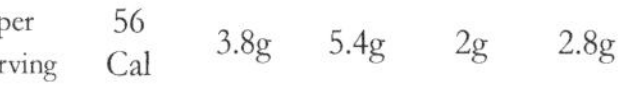
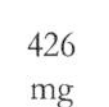

per serving	56 Cal	3.8g	5.4g	2g	2.8g		426 mg

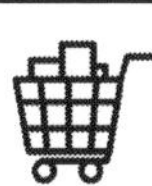

- Small squash - 1
- One teaspoon salt
- Stevia – ½ tsp.
- Water – 2 cups
- Olive oil - 12 tablespoon

1. Start by lining a rimmed baking sheet with parchment paper and preheating the oven to 425 degrees Fahrenheit.. Just enough olive oil, or approximately a half-teaspoon for each half, should be used to lightly coat the inside of the butternut squash before placing it on the pan. Salt the inside of the squash and then rub the oil all over it.
2. Grill the squash for 40 to 50 minutes, or till it is tender, with the cut side down. and cooked through (don't worry if the skin or flesh browns—good that's for flavor). The squash should be set aside for 10 minute or until it is cold enough to handle.
3. In the meantime, heat 1 tablespoon of olive oil in a large soup pot until shimmering (if your blender has a soup present, use a medium skillet to minutes dishes) Place the ingredients in your stand. Scoop the squash flesh into your blender using a big spoon. Throw away the hard skin. To the blender, add the stevia. Pour 2 cups of water into the container, being cautious not to fill it over the maximum fill line
4. Fasten the lid firmly. In order to prevent heated steam from escaping from the lid, blend on high Once your soup is thoroughly heated and incredibly creamy.
5. Stir in the final cup of water if you want to thin out your soup even further. To taste, stir in 1 to 2 tbsp. of butter or olive oil. If required, add extra salt and pepper after tasting.
6. You can pour your soup into serving dishes if it has just finished blending and is still boiling hot. If not, re-pour it into the soup pot and boil it over medium heat, stirring frequently, until it is minutes hot.

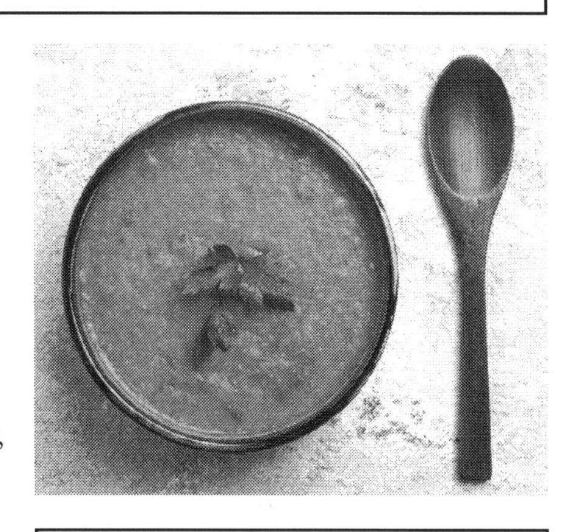

Storage:
For quick cooling, store soup in shallow containers. Soups can last up to 3 days in the fridge when covered.

Reheat:
Whether in the microwave or on the stove top, reheating soup is simple.

 4  14"  41"

6.2 Vegetable Soup

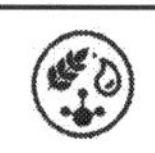 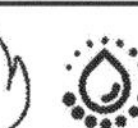 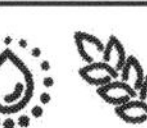 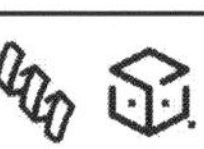 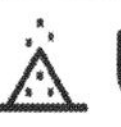

per serving	92 Cal	3.7g	14.2g	2.3g	3.1g		512 mg

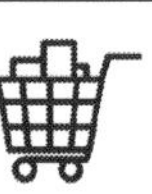

- Olive oil – 1 tbsp.
- Chopped, peeled carrots – 1 cup
- Water – 2cups
- Diced, skinned potatoes – 1 cup
- Chopped zucchini – 1 cup
- Fresh, chopped parsley – ¼ cup
- Salt
- Chopped frozen or fresh green beans - 3/4 cup

1. In a large pot, preheat the olive oil over medium-high heat..
2. After carrots, and potatoes, zucchini parsley, and water should also be added. Salt should also be added to taste.
3. Green beans are added after bringing reach a boil.
4. Once potatoes are almost totally soft, lower heat to medium-low, cover, and simmer for 20 to 30 minutes.
5. Serve hot.

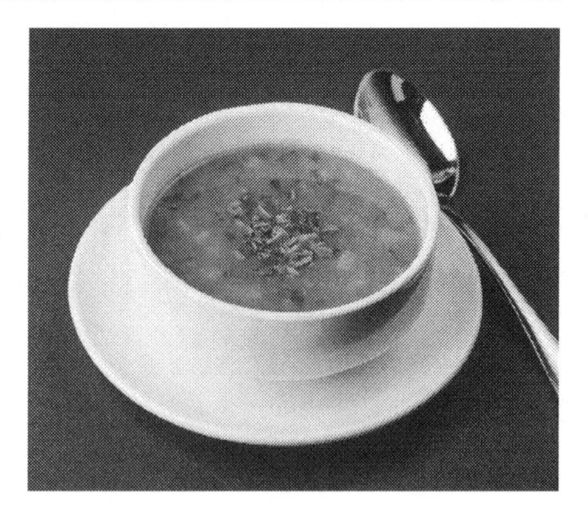

Storage:
For quick cooling, store soup in shallow containers. Soups can last up to 3 days in the fridge when covered.

Reheat:
Whether in the microwave or on the stove topp, reheating soup is simple.

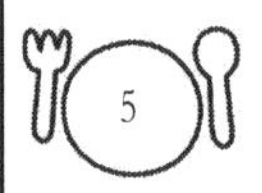 5  24"  12"

6.3 Kale and Carrot Soup

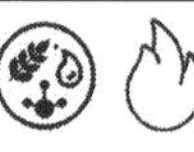 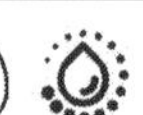 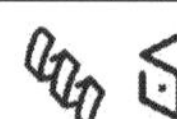 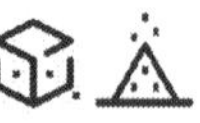 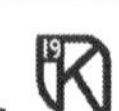

per serving	65 Cal	0g	14.3g	3g	2.7g		596 mg

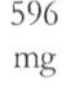

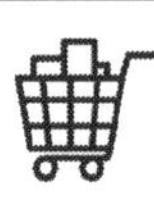

- Apple cider vinegar - ½ tablespoon
- Carrots– 2 cups
- Water – 2 cups
- Kale – 1 1/2 cups
- Fresh basil – 1/8 cup

1. Simmer the carrots in a large stockpot with a steamer insert over medium heat for 1 to 2 minutes..
2. Fill the steamer insert with the whole kale leaves, basil leaves.Place the steamer into the stockpot, cover it, and steam for 5 to 7 minutes, stirring halfway through with tongs. Eliminate sate and discard the basil. The soup will simmer again when you add the kale and vinegar. If desired, season with salt a. Just before serving, add the basil in chopped form.

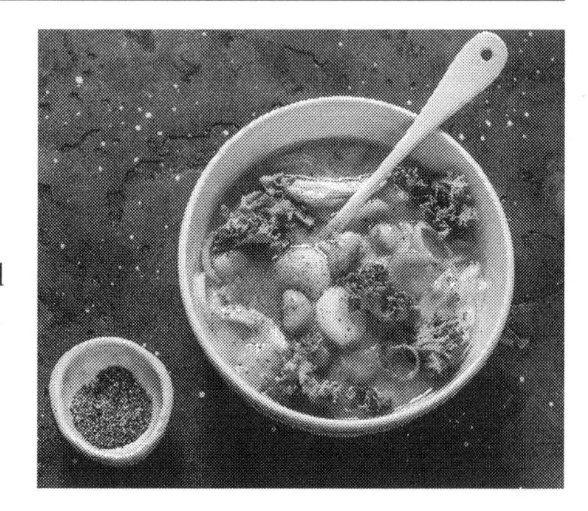

Storage:
For quick cooling, store soup in shallow containers. Soups can last up to 3 days in the fridge when covered.

Reheat:
Whether in the microwave or on the stove top, reheating soup is simple.

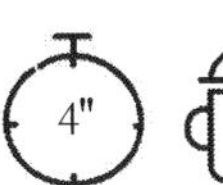

6.4 Pumpkin Soup

	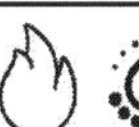	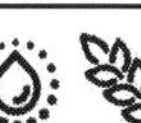	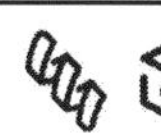	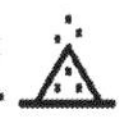	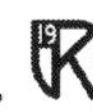
per serving	85 Cal	0.8g	20.2g	2.8g 8.3g	519 mg

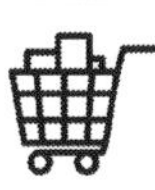

- 1 pound pumpkin
- Salt
- 3 cups of water

1. the pumpkin into 2.25"/3.0 cm pieces "slices. Remove the skin, then remove the seeds. Slice into 1.5/4 cm "chunks.
2. In a pot, combine the pumpkin, and water; the liquid will not completely cover the pumpkin. Covered, Bring to a boil, then immediately reduce heat, cover, and simmer for 10 minutes, or until pumpkin is tender.
3. Remove from heat, then puree using a stick blender until smooth .
4. Add salt to taste.
5. Pour soup into bowls.

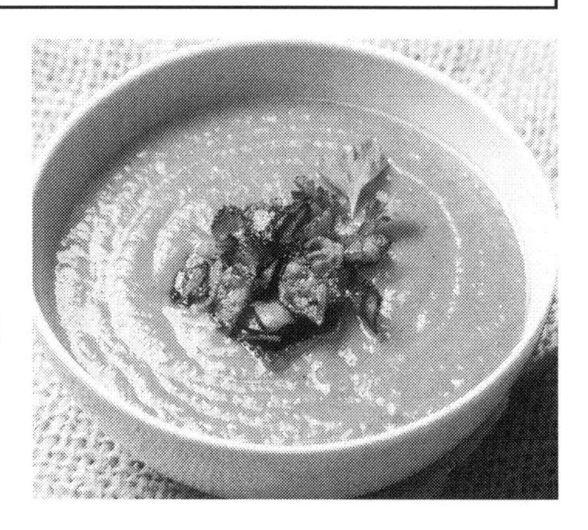

Storage:
For quick cooling, store soup in shallow containers. Soups can last up to 3 days in the fridge when covered.

Reheat:
Whether in the microwave or on the stove top, reheating soup is simple.

6.5 Zucchini Soup

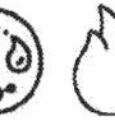	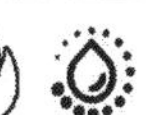		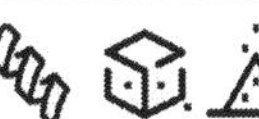	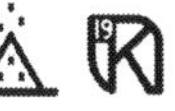
per serving	170 Cal	17.2g	5.5g 1.8g 2.6g	408 mg

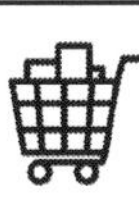

- Olive oil, 4 tbsp.
- Chopped zucchini- 1 pound
- Salt – 1 teaspoon
- Water – 2 cups
- Curry powder, 1 teaspoon

1. In a pot over medium heat, warm the olive oil. By adding the zucchini to the pot along with the water, salt, and curry powder, cook the zucchini for about 15 minutes, or until it is tender.
2. Pour soup into a blender no more than halfway full. After covering and keeping the lid on, pulse several times before blending in batches until the mixture is perfectly smooth.

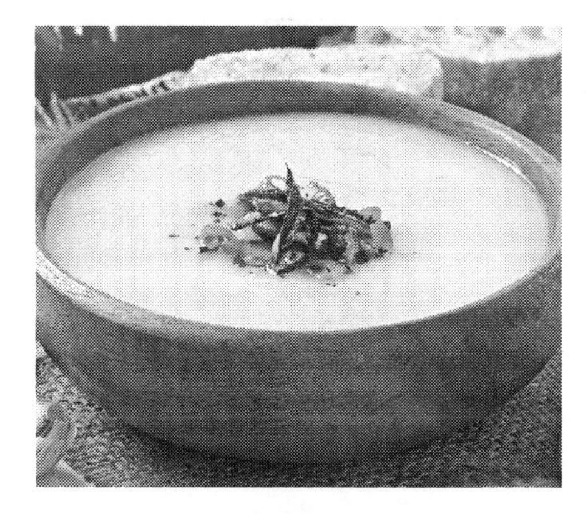

Storage:
For quick cooling, store soup in shallow containers. Soups can last up to 3 days in the fridge when covered.

Reheat:
Whether in the microwave or on the stove top, reheating soup is simple.

 5  11"  14"

6.6 Creamy Potato Kale Soup

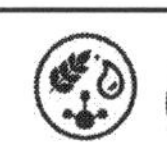 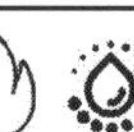 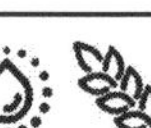 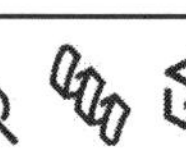 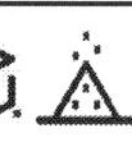 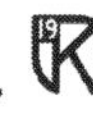

per serving	265 Cal	21.4g	18.4g	3.3g	3g		588 mg

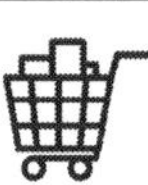

- 2-and-a-half tbsp, of olive oil
- 2 small potatoes, roughly diced after being peeled
- Water in 4 glasses
- 1 cup of chopped kale
- Coconut milk- 1 cup
- Salt to taste

1. Heat the oil in a large pot over medium-high heat. When the potatoes are golden brown, add them and simmer for an additional 5-8 minutes. Use salt to season. After cooking in the 3 cups of water for 5 to 10 minutes, the kale should soften and turn a darker green.
2. Use a strong blender to puree the soup. It takes around 2-3 minutes to completely smooth out the soup. Return the pureed soup to the pan and whisk in the milk and remaining 1 cup of water, depending on how thick you want the soup to be.

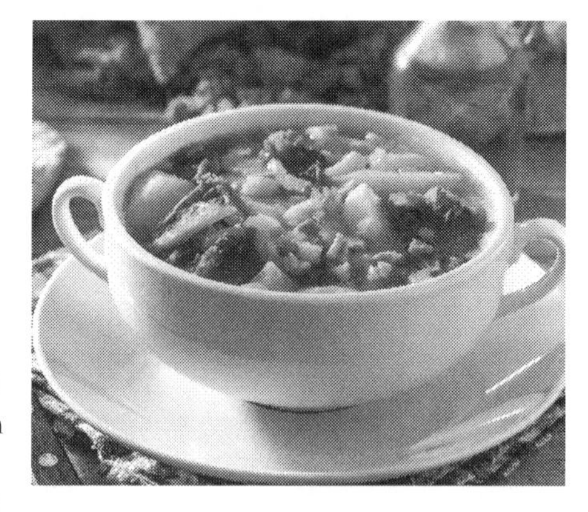

Storage:
For quick cooling, store soup in shallow containers. Soups can last up to 3 days in the fridge when covered.

Reheat:
Whether in the microwave or on the stove top, reheating soup is simple.

 5  11"  28"

6.7 Chicken Zucchini Soup

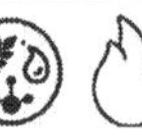 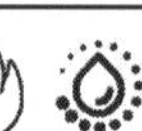 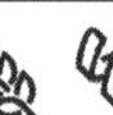 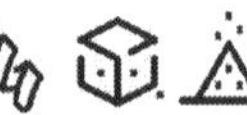 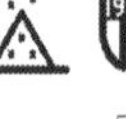 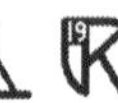

per serving	186 Cal	6.7g	5.7g	26.1g	2.9g		588 mg

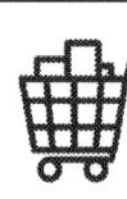

- 1 pound of skinless, boneless chicken breast
- 1 tbsp, of olive oil
- 6 cups finely diced zucchini (any seeds removed)
- 1/4 cup dried basil
- Salt, 1/2 teaspoon
- Water in 4 glasses

1. Cut the chicken into bite-sized chunks about 1/2 to 1 inch. Pour ½ tablespoon of the olive oil into a sizable stockpot and set it to medium heat. About 7 to 10 minutes later, When the chicken is no longer pink, add it and thoroughly cook it. Take out of the pot and set aside.
2. The stock pot should remain on medium heat as you add the final ½ tablespoon of olive oil to it.
3. Add water, basil, salt, and zucchini. When the zucchini is soft and tender, simmer for another 15 minutes, stirring frequently.
4. If you want any chunks or texture in your soup, take off about 2 cups of it and set them aside. Otherwise, leave it in. Blend the zucchini in the pot until it is smooth, using a blender. Stirring constantly, add the chicken and remaining zucchini back to the saucepan. Serve warm

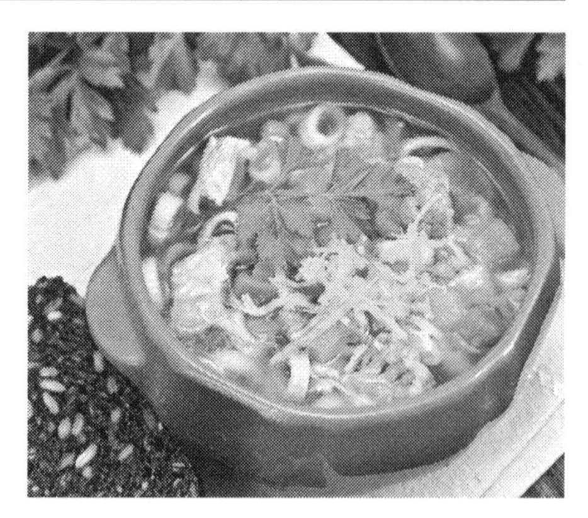

Storage:
For quick cooling, store soup in shallow containers. Soups can last up to 3 days in the fridge when covered.

Reheat:
Whether in the microwave or on the stove top, reheating soup is simple.

 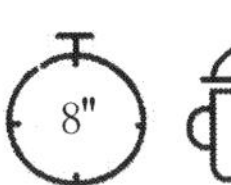 

6.8 Green Bean Soup

 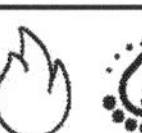 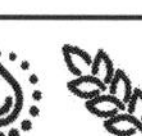 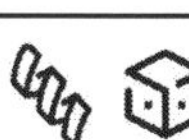 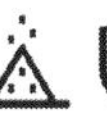 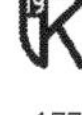

per serving	77 Cal	7.1g	3.9g	1g	0.9g		177 mg

- Water, - 2 cups
- 1 handful of cut basil leaves
- Salt
- Shelled green beans - 1 cup
- Olive oil – 1 tbsp.

1. Warm the olive oil in a small casserole over medium heat.
2. Add the beans and water. Cook the beans steadily for 7-8 minutes, or until they are very soft, after bringing to a simmer.
3. Puree the soup in a food processor or with an immersion blender. Re-simmer the soup after adding the remaining colored beans. Cook the beef for 4–5 minutes, or until it is tender.
4. If necessary, add salt. Pour into still-warm bowls and top with a few basil slices for decoration.

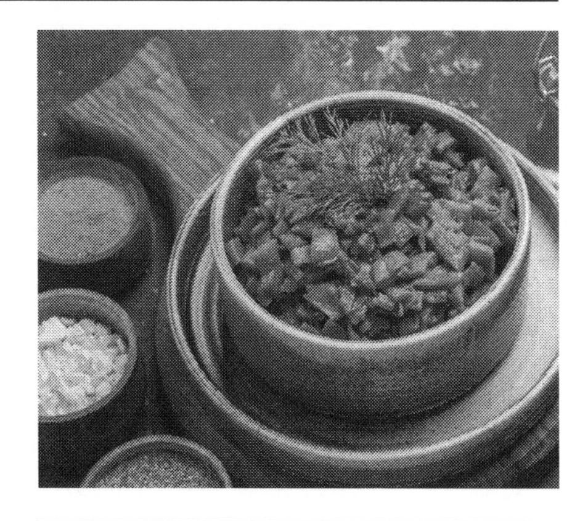

Storage:
For quick cooling, store soup in shallow containers. Soups can last up to 3 days in the fridge when covered.

Reheat:
Whether in the microwave or on the stove top, reheating soup is simple.

6.9 Fish and Vegetable Soup

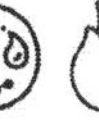   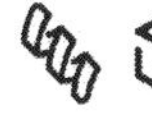 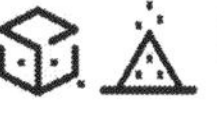 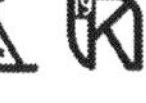

per serving	203 Cal	10.7g	5.4g	22.9g	1.9g		596 mg

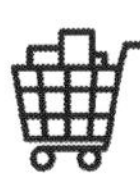

- Ingredients
- Dried oregano leaves, ¼ teaspoon
- Olive oil, ½ tablespoon
- Water – 2 cups
- Carrots, finely sliced – ½ cup
- Chopped frozen green beans – ½ cup
- Half-spoon of salt
- Dried basil leaves – 2 tbsp.
- Salmon fillets – ½ pound

1. In a Dutch oven or 3-quart saucepan, heat the oil over medium heat. After combining the remaining ingredients, add the fish last. up to a boil. With a cover on, simmer for 8 minutes over low heat.
2. Fish should now be added and cooked for 5 to 7 minutes, stirring regularly, until it flakes easily and the veggies are soft.

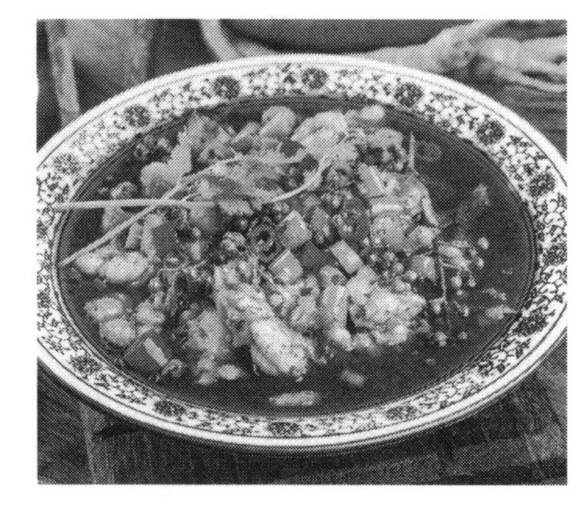

Storage:
For quick cooling, store soup in shallow containers. Soups can last up to 3 days in the fridge when covered.

Reheat:
Whether in the microwave or on the stove top, reheating soup is simple.

3
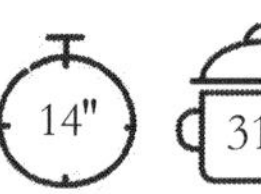
14"
31"

6.10 Broccoli Feta Soup

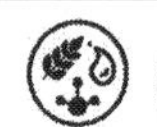
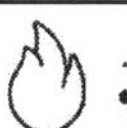
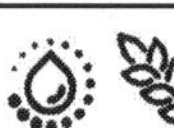
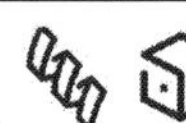
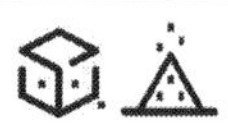

per serving	356 Cal	31.8g	12.4g	11.2g	3.8g		222 mg

- Olive oil – 1/8 cup
- Grated small carrot – ½
- Quinoa flour -8 ounces
- Water – ½ quart
- Coconut milk, 1 cup
- Grated feta cheese, 4 ounces
- Salt – ½ tsp.
- Small broccoli, cut into stems and florets.

1. Add a couple generous pinches of salt and heat a sizable pot of water until it boils. Broccoli stalks should be bright green, fork-tender, but still somewhat crunchy after 2 to 3 minutes of blanching.
2. Rinse the broccoli. About 1 cup of the florets should be scooped out and saved for the topping.
3. Clean the saucepan, then Warm the oil there over a medium heat. Put carrots in When the vegetables are soft, cook for another 4 to 5 minutes while stirring often.
4. Add the quinoa flour and stir. The flour and vegetables will combine to make a paste. After coating the veggies with the cooking liquid for one or two minutes, begin to slowly pour in the water. While pouring, constantly stir.
5. Bring the soup to a gentle simmer after all the water has been added. Add milk and all but a little amount of the blanched broccoli (for the topping). Over low heat, simmer for approximately ten minutes.
6. Blend using a blender in batches or an immersion blender, wait until the soup has stopped.
7. To the soup that has been pureed, add the grated cheese, salt, and stir until the cheese has melted. Taste the soup and season with additional salt to your satisfaction.
8. Pour the soup into dishes and top each one with additional cheese and some of the saved broccoli.

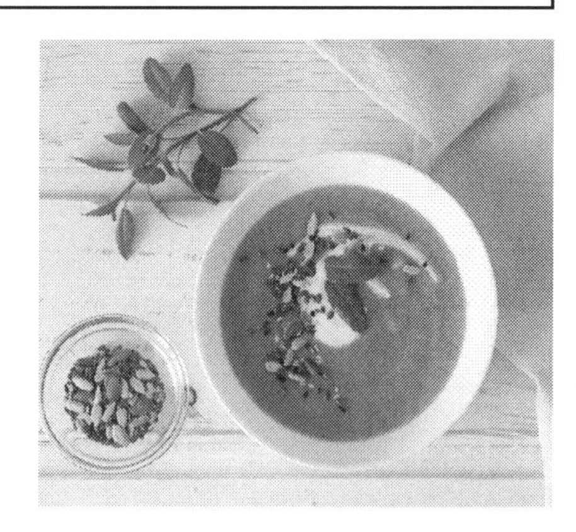

Storage:
For quick cooling, store soup in shallow containers. Soups can last up to 3 days in the fridge when covered.

Reheat:
Whether in the microwave or on the stove top, reheating soup is simple.

CHAPTER 7

FISH AND SHELLFISH

 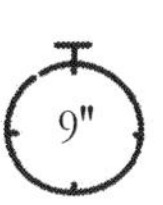 

7.1 Salmon and Vegetable Quinoa

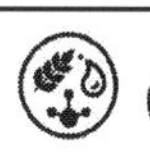 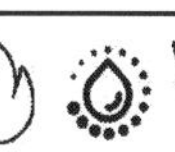  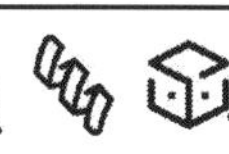 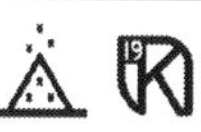

per serving	381 Cal	11.7g	37g	35.1g	3.6g	979 mg

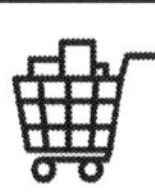

- Quinoa
- Kosher salt – ¼ tsp.
- a one tiny cucumber, sliced and seeded
- two basil leaves,
- one lemon's thinly sliced zest
- Quinoa, - ½ cup
- Salmon
- kosher salt, 1/4 teaspoon
- Salmon fillets - 4 fillets
- 4 slices of lemon
- 1/8 cup freshly chopped parsley

1. Bring ½ cup of quinoa, In a medium saucepan with a lid, bring one cup of water and one-half teaspoon of salt to a boil.
2. When the quinoa is frothy and light, cook it for about 20 minutes or as directed on the package, covered and at a simmer.
3. Before serving, turn off the heat and let the dish sit covered for at least five minutes.
4. Combine the cucumbers, basil, and lemon zest just before serving. Make the salmon in the meanwhile.
5. Foil should be used to line a sheet pan or glass dish, and nonstick cooking spray or olive oil should be used to lightly coat it.
6. Place the salmon fillets in the pan, then sprinkle roughly a half teaspoon of the salt mixture over the surface of each fillet.
7. Put the lemon wedges along the pan's outside edges.
8. Salmon should be done and readily flaked apart with a fork after 8 to 10 minutes of broiling on high with the rack in the lowest third of the oven.
9. With roasted lemon wedges and vegetarian quinoa, garnish with parsley.

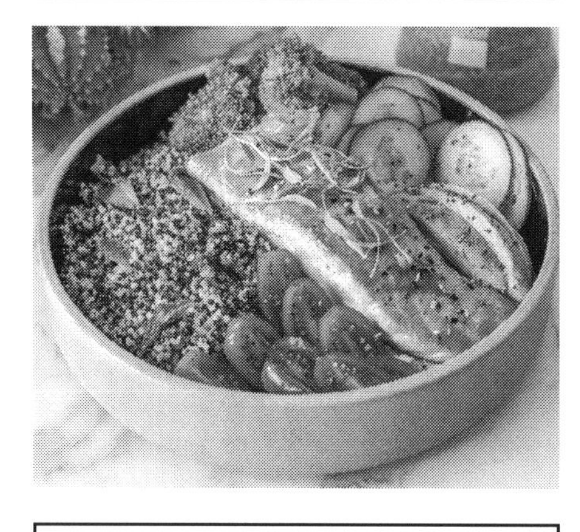

Storage:
Wrap securely with heavy-duty aluminum foil or freezer wrap and freeze in closed, airtight containers or freezer bags..

Reheat:
Put the fish on a rimmed pan and reheat it in a preheated oven set to 275 degrees Fahrenheit. Warm for 15 minutes, or until the inside reaches 125–130 F.

 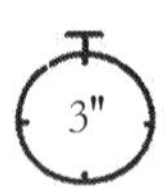 

7.2 Baked Salmon

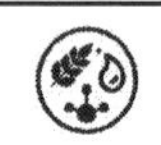 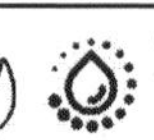 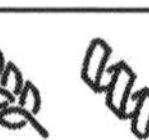 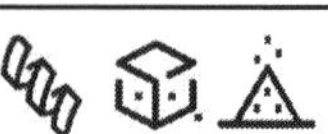 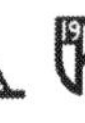 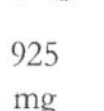

per serving	491 Cal	35.2g	3.2g	44.4g	0.8g	925 mg

- 1 finely sliced lemon
- Salmon fillet -1 1/2 pounds
- Salt
- Olive oil – 3 tbsp.
- Stevia – 1 tsp.
- Basil leaves – 1 tbsp.
- One teaspoon dried oregano
- Fresh parsley, chopped, as a garnish
- Cooking spray

1. 350 degrees in the oven. Grease a large baking sheet with a rim with cooking spray. In the center of the foil, put a layer of lemon slices.
2. Place lemon slices on top of salmon that has been salt and peppered on both sides.
3. In a small bowl, mix the oil, stevia, basil, and oregano. The salmon should be covered with the liquid, then foil. Bake the salmon for about 25 minutes, or until it is completely cooked. Set the oven to broil and wait two minutes, or until the butter mixture has thickened.
4. Before serving, garnish with parsley.

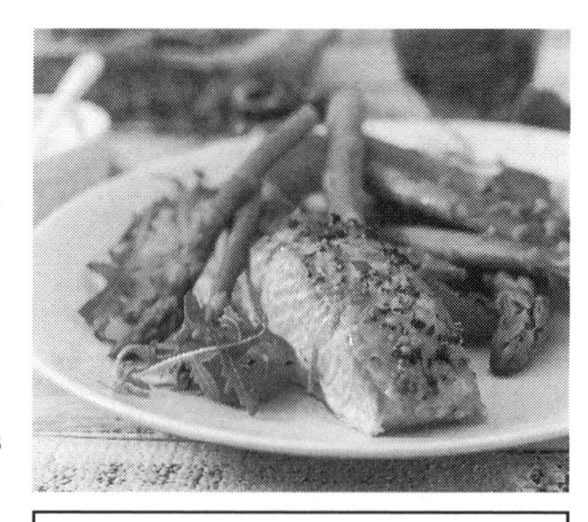

Storage:
Wrap securely with heavy-duty aluminum foil or freezer wrap and freeze in closed, airtight containers or freezer bags

Reheat:
Put the fish on a rimmed pan and reheat it in a preheated oven set to 275 degrees Fahrenheit. Warm for 15 minutes, or until the inside reaches 125–130 F.

 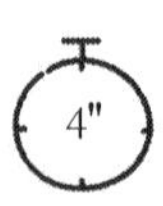 

7.3 Grilled Salmon

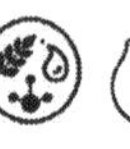 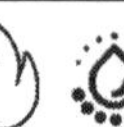 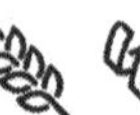 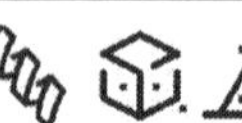 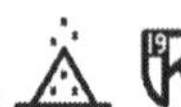 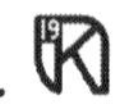

per serving	255 Cal	13.3g	1.1g	33g	0g	655 mg

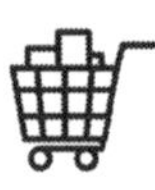

- 4 salmon fillets (6 ounces)
- Salt
- Whole grain mustard, 4 tbsp,
- 1/4 cup stevia
- 2 teaspoons olive oil
- Fresh cilantro leaves, half a teaspoon

1. Use salt to season the fish all over, mustard, stevia, oil, and cilantro should all be combined in a small bowl. Salmon should be covered in the mixture.
2. For several minutes, heat the grill pan over medium-high heat until your hand can't be held directly over it. If the fillets have skin, place it skin-side up on the grill pan. For the grill pan marks to nicely sear in, leave them in place for one minute.

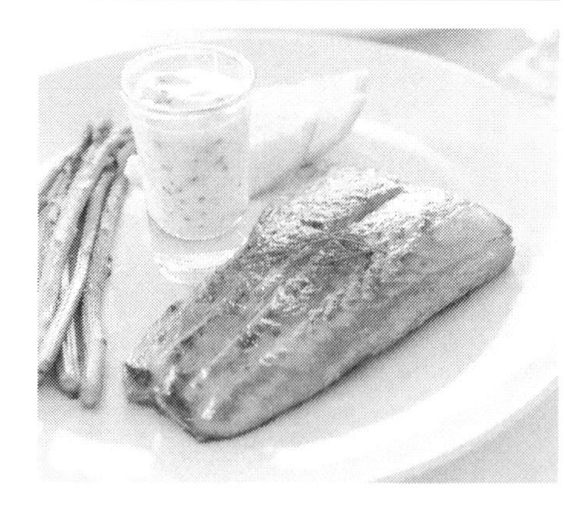

Storage:
Wrap securely with heavy-duty foil or freezer wrap and freeze in closed, airtight containers or freezer bags..

Reheat:
Reheat the fish in an oven that has been preheated to 275 degrees Fahrenheit by placing it on a rimmed pan. Warm for 15 minutes or until the internal temperature is between 125 and 130 F.

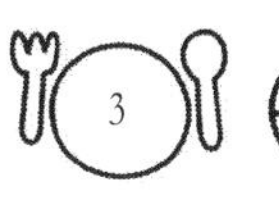

7.4 Tuscan Salmon

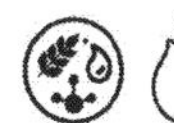
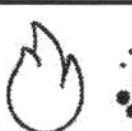
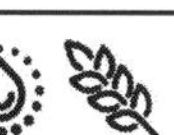
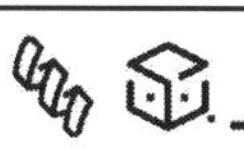
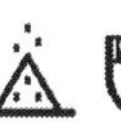

per serving	363 Cal	21.7g	7.2g	37.3g	0.9g	979 mg

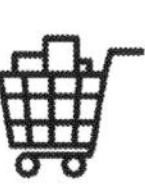

- Herbs, such as basil and parsley, for garnish – ¼ cup
- Olive oil – 1 tbsp.
- Freshly grated feta - 1/4 cup
- Salmon fillets, 2
- Salt
- Serving slices of lemon
- Kale – 1 cup

1. In a large skillet, heat the oil to medium-high heat. the salmon with salt all over. When oil is shimmering but not smoking, add salmon skin side up and cook for about 6 minutes, until fully browned. Before rotating, cook for two more minutes. Put on a plate.
2. Add oil after lowering the heat to medium. Add salt to taste. Add kale after cooking until tomatoes are starting to burst. Cook just until the spinach starts to wilt.
3. After bringing the mixture to a simmer, add the feta and herbs. Simmer for three minutes, or until the sauce has slightly reduced, on low heat.
4. Put the salmon back in the skillet and top with sauce. Simmer for a further 3 minutes or until salmon is thoroughly done.
5. Before serving, garnish with additional herbs and squeeze lemon over top.

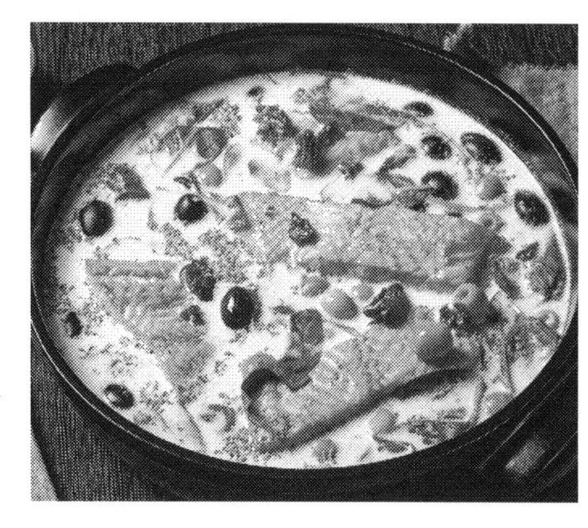

Storage:
Wrap securely with heavy-duty aluminum foil or freezer wrap and freeze in closed, airtight containers or freezer bags..

Reheat:
Put the fish on a rimmed pan and reheat it in a preheated oven set to 275 degrees Fahrenheit. Warm for 15 minutes, or until the inside reaches 125–130 F.

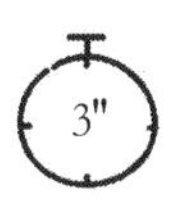

7.5 Baked Cod

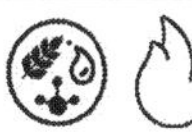
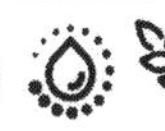
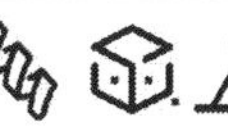

per serving	203 Cal	8.6g	0.3g	31.7g	0.2g	16 mg

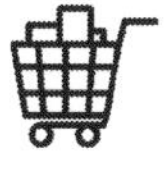

- Salt – 1/8 tsp.
- Cod -2 fillets
- Lemon juice – 1-1/2 tbsp.
- Olive oil – 8 tbsp.
- Dried oregano – ½ tsp

1. Place the fish in a 13 x 9-inch, non-oiled baking dish. In a small bowl, combine the oil, lemon juice, oregano and salt. Apply the mixture to the fillets. As a garnish, add the oregano.
2. Bake fish for 10 to 15 minutes at 425 degrees, or until it just begins to flake easily when tested with a fork.

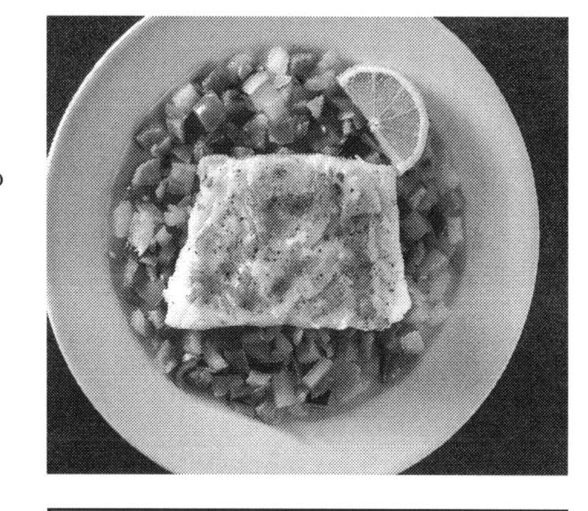

Storage:
Wrap securely with heavy-duty aluminum foil or freezer wrap and freeze in closed, airtight containers or freezer bags..

Reheat:
Put the fish on a rimmed pan and reheat it in a preheated oven set to 275 degrees Fahrenheit. Warm for 15 minutes, or until the inside reaches 125–130 F.

7.6 Quick Shrimp Stir Fry

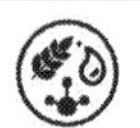	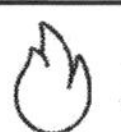	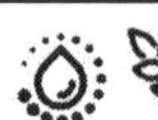	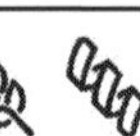	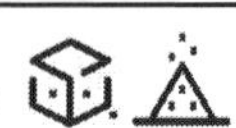	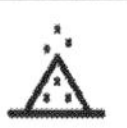	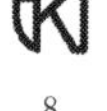
per serving	133 Cal	7g	2.5g	21.3g	0.1g	8 mg

- 1/2 pound of huge, deveined shrimp (tail on or off)
- Slice of lemon
- Salt
- chopped cilantro or parsley as a garnish
- Dried oregano -1/4 tsp
- Olive oil, 1 tbsp.

1. Either preheat the broiler or the oven to 400 degrees Fahrenheit.
2. Thaw any frozen shrimp.
3. To dry, pat the shrimp. Toss the shrimp with the olive oil, oregano and salt in a medium bowl.
4. Baked technique: Use parchment paper to cover a baking sheet. Put the shrimp in an equal layer on a baking pan. Depending on the size of the shrimp. Bake the shrimp on the baking sheet for 4 to 6 minutes, or until they are plump and opaque.
5. Shrimp should be spread out evenly on a baking sheet for the broiler method. Broil the baking sheet for 3 to 6 minutes, or until the food is moist and opaque.
6. For even cooking, turn the tray as necessary.
7. Sprinkle freshly cut parsley or cilantro on top, spritz with fresh lemon juice from lemon wedges, and serve it for right away.

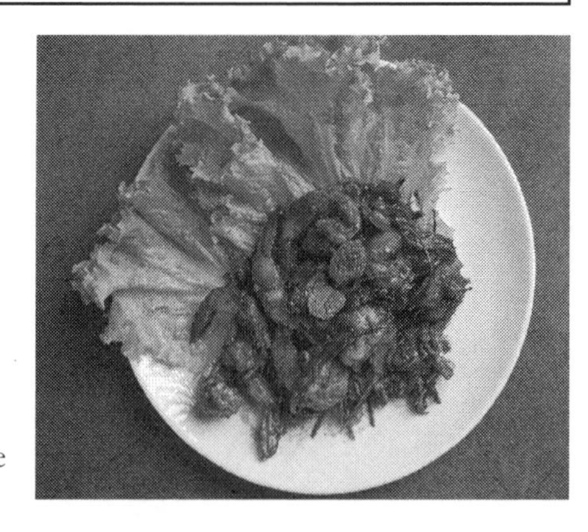

Storage:
While it will typically continue to be safe to eat after that, properly maintained, frozen cooked shrimp will maintain its finest quality for around

Reheat:
Put the fish on a rimmed pan and reheat it in a preheated oven set to 300degrees Fahrenheit. Warm for 15 minutes, or until the inside reaches 125–130 F.

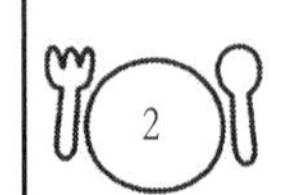

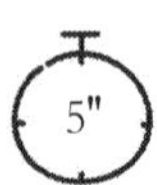

7.7 Shrimp Fried Quinoa

	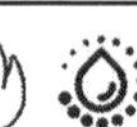				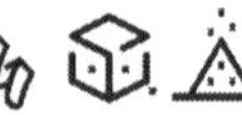	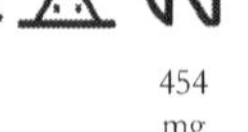	
per serving	487 Cal	25.3g	28.5g	36.4g	3.1g		454 mg

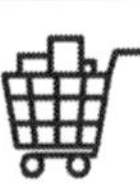

- Medium-sized shrimp 1/2 pound
- Carrots 1
- Chopped green cabbage, half a cup
- Divided 2.5 tbsp, of sesame oil
- 2 eggs
- Green beans, 1/2 cup
- Cooked quinoa, two cups
- Salt 1 tsp.

1. Defrost the shrimp.
2. Carrots should be peeled and then diced. Chop the cabbage if using.
3. To dry, pat the shrimp. 2 tbsp, of sesame oil are heated on medium high in a large skillet. With tongs, add the shrimp and fry them for about a minute on each side, until just opaque and cooked through. Due to the fact that you'll be adding them to the quinoa later, they may be little undercooked.
4. Add a half-teaspoon of salt. Take out and place in a basin.
5. Heat 1 tbsp, of the sesame oil to medium high in a big skillet or wok. For two minutes, sauté carrots.
6. Sauté for 2 minutes after adding the cabbage. For one minute, stir in the quinoas, green beans, and remaining 1/2 teaspoon salt.
7. Quinoa should be pushed aside. Add one more tablespoon of oil. Add a pinch of salt and scramble the eggs for 1 to 2 minutes, or until they are fully cooked.
8. Serve warm.

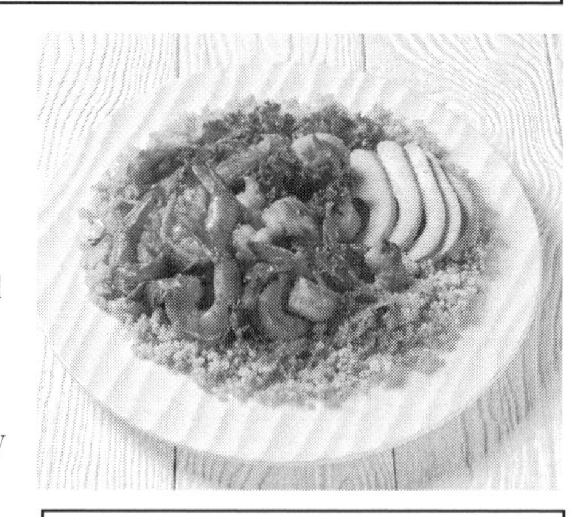

Storage:
While it will typically continue to be safe to eat after that, properly maintained, frozen cooked shrimp will maintain its finest quality for around 10 to 12 months in the freezer.

Reheat:
Put the fish on a rimmed pan and reheat it in a preheated oven set to 300 degrees Fahrenheit. Warm for 15 minutes, or until the inside reaches 125–130 F

 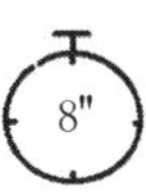 

7.8 Lemony zucchini noodles with cod

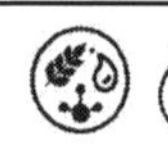 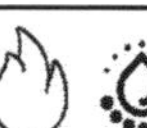 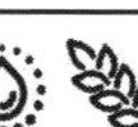 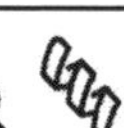 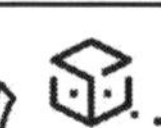 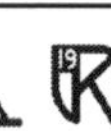

per serving	240 Cal	8.6g	6.5g	34.7g	3.1g		841 mg

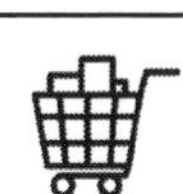

- Cod, 20 ounces
- Salt to taste
- Two tbsp, of olive oil

Noodles:

- Olive oil, 1 tbsp
- One teaspoon of lemon juice
- Zucchini noodles, 24 ounces (zoodles)
- Salt as desired
- 1/2 cup chopped Italian parsley
- Lemon zest, 2 teaspoons,

1. Turn on the oven to 375°F (or toaster oven)
2. In a medium skillet over medium heat, warm the oil. Cod needs to be dried, salted. Cook cod both sides in a pan until brown.
3. After all sides are brown, place fish in the warm oven. (between 3 and 6 minutes, depending on how thick the incision is)
4. Take a large skillet with additional oil is heated over medium heat.
5. Add zucchini noodles in skillet. The noodles should soften after being sautéed for about 4 minutes. Lemon zest, fresh parsley, and lemon juice should be added.
6. After tasting for salt and lemon, adjust as necessary. Divide among five bowls, then top with the cod.

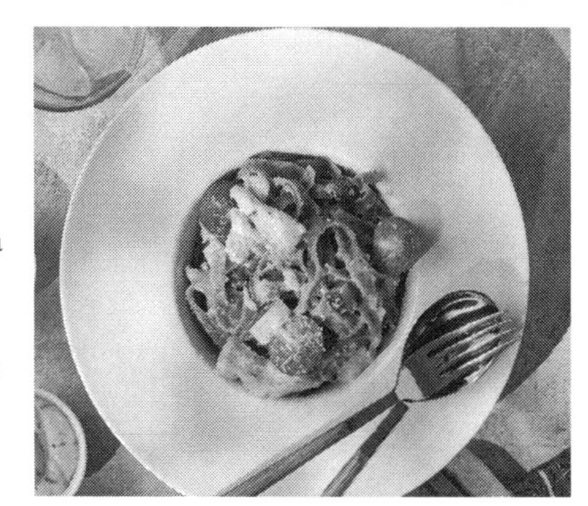

Storage:
While it will typically continue to be safe to eat after that, properly maintained, frozen cooked shrimp will maintain its finest quality for around 10 to 12 months in the freezer.

Reheat:
Put the fish on a rimmed pan and reheat it in a preheated oven set to 300 degrees Fahrenheit. Warm for 15 minutes, or until the inside reaches 125–130 F

7.9 Ceviche

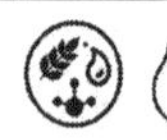   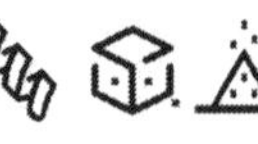 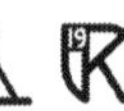 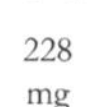

per serving	128 Cal	3.2g	9.6g	16.9g	2.9g		228 mg

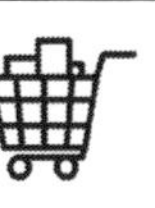

- Lime juice - 6 tbsp.
- Salt – ½ tsp.
- Fresh fish, such as salmon or cod, cut into cubes of 1/2 inch. – ½ pound
- Tomato -1
- Cilantro, - 6 tbsp.
- Cucumber – ½ cup
- Olive oil, 1/2 tablespoon (optional)

1. Place the fish in a basin with the salt, lime juice.
2. Add the olive oil, tomatoes, cucumber, and cilantro. Before serving, let the food marinate for at least 30 minutes in the fridge (45-60 minutes is ideal). The longer you marinate the fish, the stiffer and more "cooked" it becomes.
3. Before serving, taste the cuisine and adjust the salt.

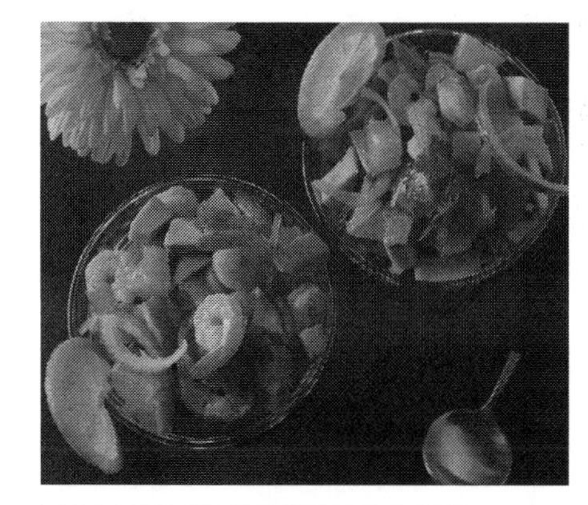

Storage:
While it will typically continue to be safe to eat after that, properly maintained, frozen cooked shrimp will maintain its finest quality for around 10 to 12 months in the freezer.

Reheat:
Put the fish on a rimmed pan and reheat it in a preheated oven set to 300 degrees Fahrenheit. Warm for 15 minutes, or until the inside reaches 125–130 F

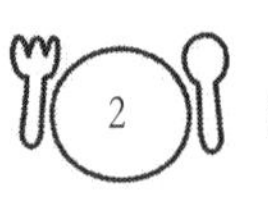 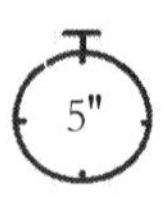 

7.10 Caramelized Salmon

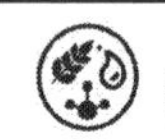 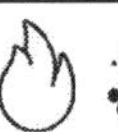 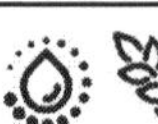 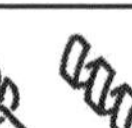 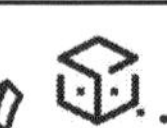 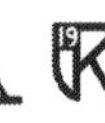

  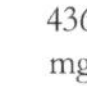

per serving	210 Cal	14g	0g	22g	0g		436 mg

- Stevia – 4 tbsp.
- Salt – ½ tsp.
- Salmon -2 fillets
- Olive oil – 2 tbsp.

1. Combine the salt and stevia in a small bowl. Spread the stevia-salt mixture over the entire surface of the salmon after dipping each fillet into the bowl.
2. Heat a small amount of olive oil in a large non-stick skillet over medium heat. Once the oil is hot, add the salmon to the pan with the skin side down and cook for about 5 minutes.
3. Simply drain it off or spoon it out of the pan if you're concerned about the burnt stevia in the pan (or if there's too much oil or liquid). Reduce the heat if there is a lot of oil splattering
4. Carefully flip each salmon fillet. Keep the skin on there (keeping the skin on makes the fillets more cohesive) and sauté for an additional 2-3 minutes. If the fillet is thick enough, flip to the side and sauté each side for an additional two to three minutes.
5. Turn the broiler on at 450 degrees. Each salmon fillet should have a teaspoon or two of the additional stevia /salt mixture sprinkled on top of it. From the stove top, place the pan in the oven. Broil the salmon for 5 to 10 minutes, monitoring to make sure it's not burning in between. As long as the salmon's tops seem golden brown, it doesn't matter whether the sugar in the pan appears to have burned. When the salmon is done cooking, take it out of the oven and let it cool down.
6. allow to cool for a while . Before eating, carefully peel off the skin; it should come off very easily despite being completely caramelized with sugar and being very dark.

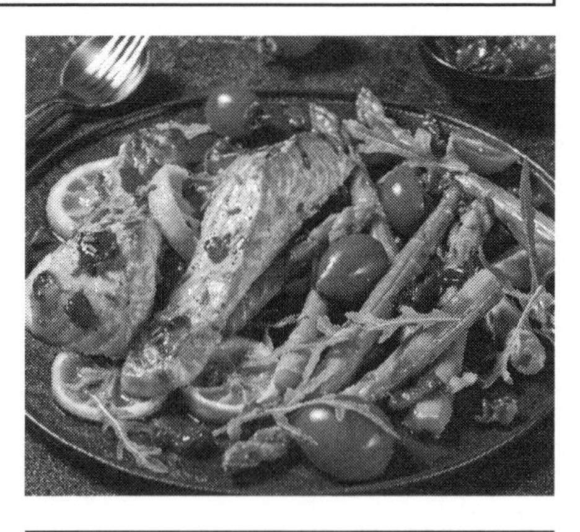

Storage:

While it will typically continue to be safe to eat after that, properly maintained, frozen cooked shrimp will maintain its finest quality for around 10 to 12 months in the freezer.

Reheat:

Put the fish on a rimmed pan and reheat it in a preheated oven set to 300 degrees Fahrenheit. Warm for 15 minutes, or until the inside reaches 125–130 F

 1  22"  13"

7.11 Herb-Roasted Salmon

 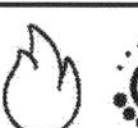 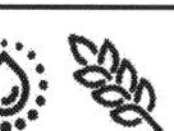  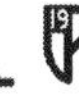

per serving | 396 Cal | 24.9g | 12.1g | 34.9g | 5g | 955 mg

- Salmon – 1 fillet
- Lemon, juiced and zest – ½
- salt, to taste
- Extra virgin olive oil – 1-1/2 tbsp.
- Parsley – 1/8 cup
- Potato - 1

Bitter Greens With Citrus Dressing

- Basil leaves - 8
- Kale – ½ cup
- Parsley – ¼ cup
- Orange, juiced and zest – ¼ cup
- Lemon, juiced and zest – ¼ cup
- Whole grain mustard - 1 tsp
- Olive oil - 6 tbsp.
- salt, kosher, to taste

1. Oven temperature: 425 °F. Sea salt and lemon zest should be mixed together with your fingers in a small bowl. Put the potatoes in a single layer and mix with 1 tablespoon of the olive oil on a big baking sheet. Take the baking sheet out of the oven after 25 minutes of roasting, then toss the potatoes with the lemon-salt mixture. Once again, roast the potatoes for 5 more minutes, or until they are golden brown and easily pierced by a sharp knife. Transfer half of the potatoes to a container for the potato salad.
2. Season salmon fillets with salt as the potatoes cook. Combine the basil, parsley, and last tablespoon of olive oil in a medium bowl.
3. In a small baking dish, arrange the salmon fillets and sprinkle with the herb mixture. The fish will be almost totally cooked after roasting for 10 minutes. After removing the dish from the oven, it should be foil-wrapped and given ten minutes to stand.
4. To make the citrus dressing, mix the lemon and orange juice, mustard, and olive oil, in a small bowl. To taste, add salt .
5. In a medium bowl, combine the kale basil , and parsley leaves. Drizzle with half of the dressing. Keep the remaining dressing aside for the recipe's green salad. Toss in salt and coat.
6. Place a salmon fillet and some lemon juice on each plate as needed. Put the dressed salad on one tray and the potatoes on the other.

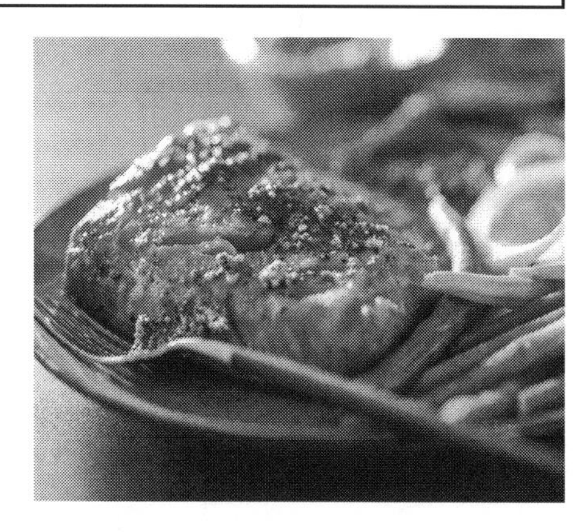

Storage:
While it will typically continue to be safe to eat after that, properly maintained, frozen cooked shrimp will maintain its finest quality for around 10 to 12 months in the freezer.

Reheat:
Put the fish on a rimmed pan and reheat it in a preheated oven set to 300 degrees Fahrenheit. Warm for 15 minutes, or until the inside reaches 125–130 F

3 | 14" | 23"

7.12 Baked salmon with green beans

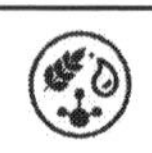 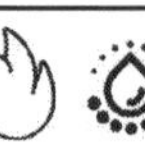  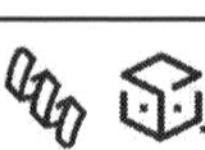 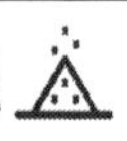 

per serving	213 Cal	5g	1.2g	39g	0.2g		436 mg

- Salt - 1/2 tsp.
- Cilantro
- 1/4 cup water
- Cod -3/4 pounds.
- Olive oil,- ½ tbsp.
- Thyme -1 tsp.
- Lemon, -1 tsp
- Green beans, one-half of a large bunch.
- Olive oil - 1 tbsp.
- The zest of one lemon

1. Heat the oven to 400 F.
2. Cod slices need to be chopped and dried. Toss to coat evenly in a bowl with the olive oil, salt, cilantro, and zest. Set aside.
3. Heat 1 tablespoon of olive oil over medium heat in a Dutch oven, cast iron pan, or oven-proof skillet, add water, lemon zest, salt, and stir.
4. After stirring, add the green beans and cook them for an additional two minutes, or until they turn a beautiful green color. If the mixture appears dry, add a little more water; you want to have about 1/4 inch of liquid in the bottom of the pan.
5. Put the fish in the pan and use a spatula to cover it with any marinade that is still on it. Bake the fish in the oven for 10-15 minutes, depending on thickness.
6. Mix together two bowls. Top with a lemon wedge and thyme leaf.

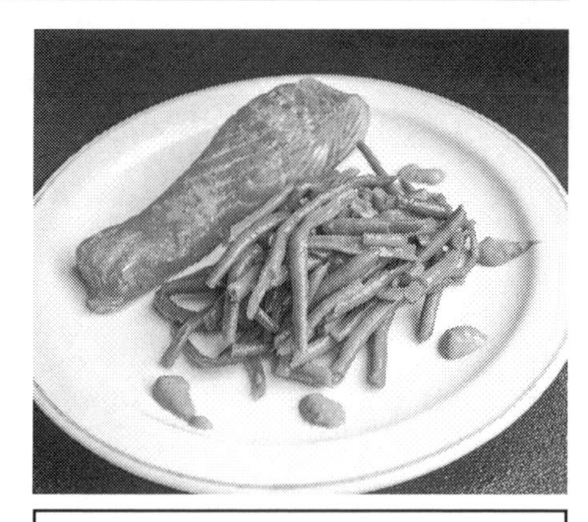

Storage:
While it will typically continue to be safe to eat after that, properly maintained, frozen cooked shrimp will maintain its finest quality for around 10 to 12 months in the freezer.

Reheat:
Put the fish on a rimmed pan and reheat it in a preheated oven set to 300 degrees Fahrenheit. Warm for 15 minutes, or until the inside reaches 125–130 F

 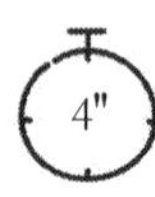 

3 | 4" | 18"

7.13 Lemon Shrimp

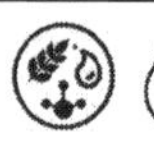 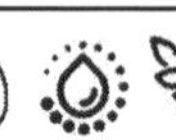 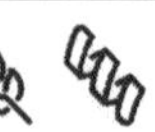 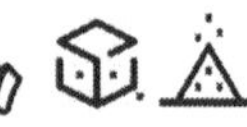 

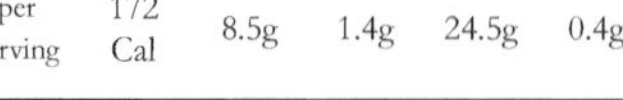

per serving	172 Cal	8.5g	1.4g	24.5g	0.4g		21 mg

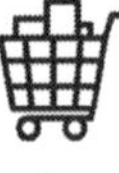

- Olive oil – 1 tbsp.
- Shrimp -1/2 pound
- Juice from 1 lemon and 1/2 lemon, thinly sliced.
- Salt
- 1/9 cup water
- Parsley, freshly chopped, as a garnish

1. Heat ½ tbsp. olive oil in a large skillet over medium heat. Salt to taste before adding the shrimp, lemon slices . About 3 minutes per side, cook shrimp, tossing periodically, until pink and opaque.
2. Water, lemon juice, and the remaining olive oil are added when the heat is turned off. Before serving, add salt and a parsley garnish.

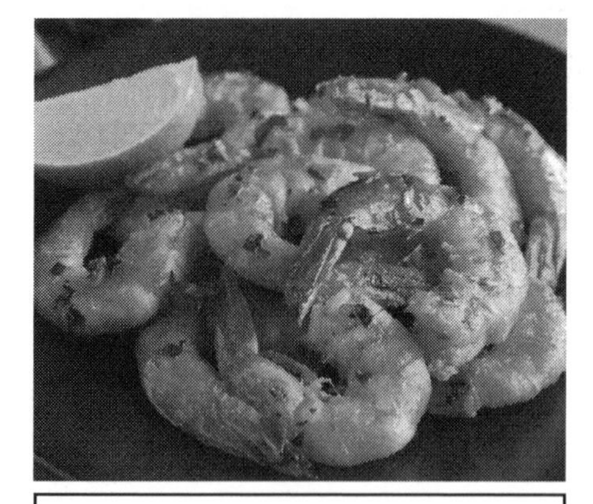

Storage:
While it will typically continue to be safe to eat after that, properly maintained, frozen cooked shrimp will maintain its finest quality for around 10 to 12 months in the freezer.

Reheat:
Put the fish on a rimmed pan and reheat it in a preheated oven set to 300degrees Fahrenheit. Warm for 15 minutes, or until the inside reaches 125–130 F

7.14 Spicy Grilled Shrimp

 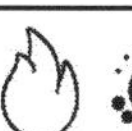 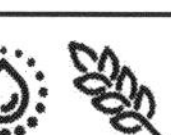 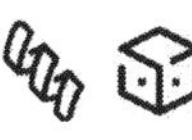 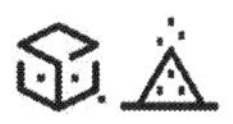 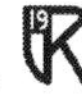

per serving	165 Cal	4.7g	3.6g	28.5g	0.3g	15 mg

- One tablespoon of lemon juice
- Half-teaspoon of salt
- Peeled and deveined 1 pound of large shrimp,
- 4 lemon wedges for garnish.
- Olive oil, 1 tbsp

1. Grill at a medium temperature.
2. To create a paste, combine lemon juice, salt and olive oil.
3. Mix the shrimp, paste, and oil in a large bowl and toss to coat the shrimp completely.
4. Give the grill grate a little oil. Grill shrimp for 2 to 3 minutes on each side, or until opaque. Sufficient for after transferring to a serving plate and adding lemon wedges as a garnish.

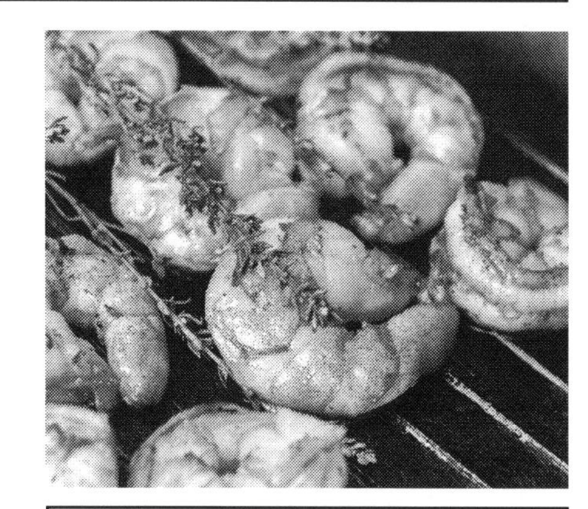

Storage:
While it will typically continue to be safe to eat after that, properly maintained, frozen cooked shrimp will maintain its finest quality for around 10 to 12 months in the freezer.

Reheat:
Put the fish on a rimmed pan and reheat it in a preheated oven set to 300degrees Fahrenheit. Warm for 15 minutes, or until the inside reaches 125–130 F

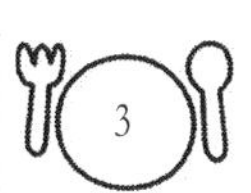

7.15 Lemon Scallops

 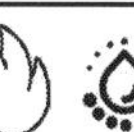 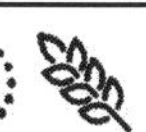 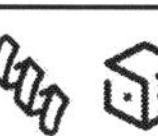 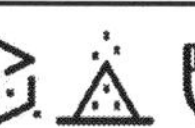 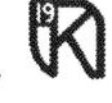

per serving	490 Cal	29.7g	9g	48.5g	0.1g	6 mg

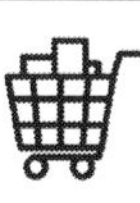

- Olive oil - 6 tbsp
- Scallops -1 lb.
- Lemon juice fresh – 1 tbsp.
- Salt – ½ tsp.

1. In a large skillet over medium-high heat, heat olive oil.. Scallops should be added and cooked for a few minutes on one side before being turned over and cooked until opaque and firm.
2. Transfer scallops to a dish, then combine oil with salt, and lemon juice. To Sufficient for, drizzle sauce over the scallops.

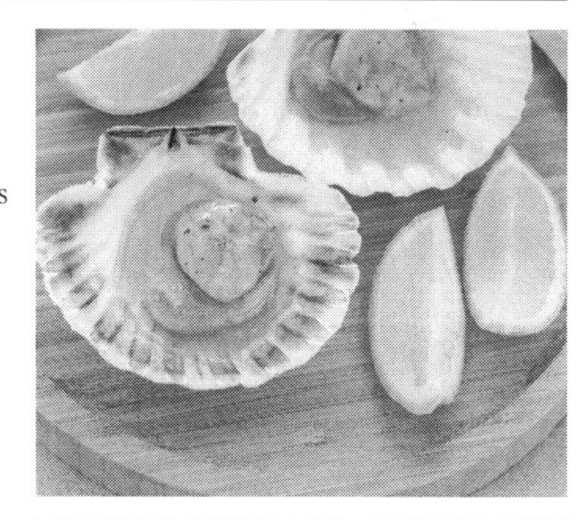

Storage:
While it will typically continue to be safe to eat after that, properly maintained, frozen cooked shrimp will maintain its finest quality for around 10 to 12 months in the freezer.

Reheat:
Put the fish on a rimmed pan and reheat it in a preheated oven set to 300degrees Fahrenheit. Warm for 15 minutes, or until the inside reaches 125–130 F

CHAPTER 8

SIDES RECIPES

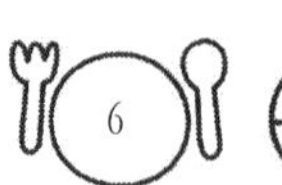
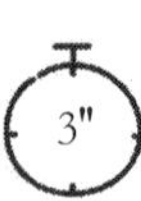

6 | 3" | 26"

8.1 Crispy Potatoes

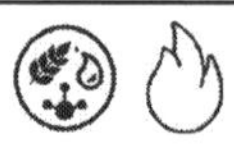
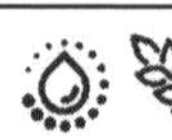
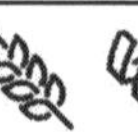
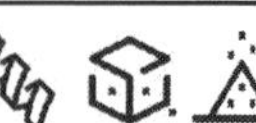
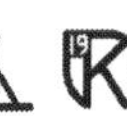
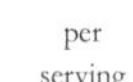
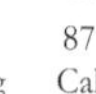
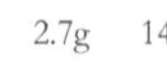
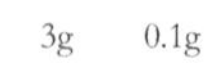

per serving	87 Cal	2.7g	14.5g	3g	0.1g		474 mg

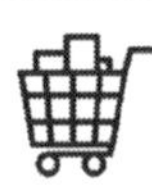

- a half-pound of young potatoes
- a tablespoon of garlic-infused oil
- salt
- serving slice of lemon
- parsley, freshly chopped, as a garnish
- 2 tbsp olive oil

1. In a large basin, combine the potatoes and a tablespoon of garlic infused oil. To taste, add salt.
2. Heat 2 tbsp, of olive oil in a 10- to 12-inch cast iron pan over medium heat until shimmering. Add the potatoes and arrange them in a single layer, cut-side down. When the potatoes are well covered with a lid, it should take around 20 minutes for the bottoms to get golden brown.
3. Remove the cover and use tongs to flip each piece to the other cut side. Cook uncovered over medium-high heat for 5 to 10 minutes more, turning the pieces as necessary, until the second side is golden brown.
4. Serve with lemon and parsley.

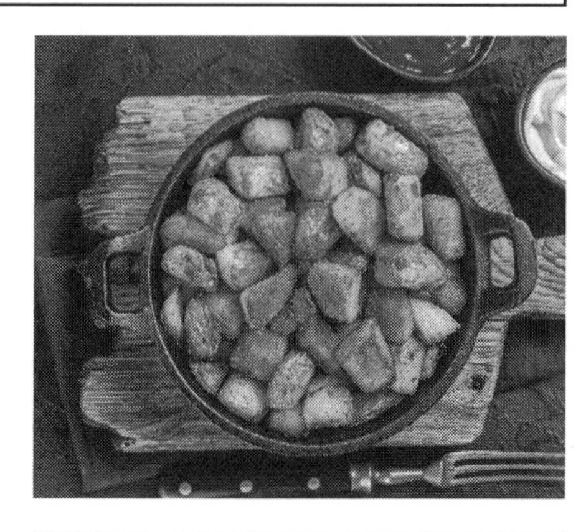

Storage:
Allow to totally cool, then wrap each one in foil or plastic wrap before putting them in an airtight freezer bag and freezing for up to three months.

Reheat:
Twice-baked potatoes can be thawed in the fridge or heated up from frozen in the oven or microwave

8.2 Roasted Broccoli

 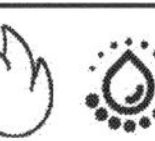 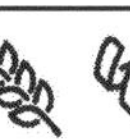 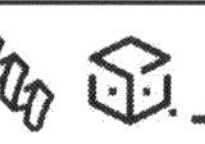 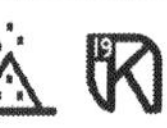

per serving	168 Cal	14.2g	10.2g	3.8g	4.6g	581 mg

- Kosher salt, 1 tsp.
- Broccoli - 1
- Olive oil, 3 tbsp.

1. To whisk eggs, simply use a fork. and include in the Set the oven to 425°F. broccoli, olive oil, kosher salt, should all be combined in a big bowl.
2. Spread the broccoli out on a sheet tray in a single layer.. When the edges of the broccoli florets have browned, roast it for 25 to 30 minutes, stirring halfway through. Sufficient for after

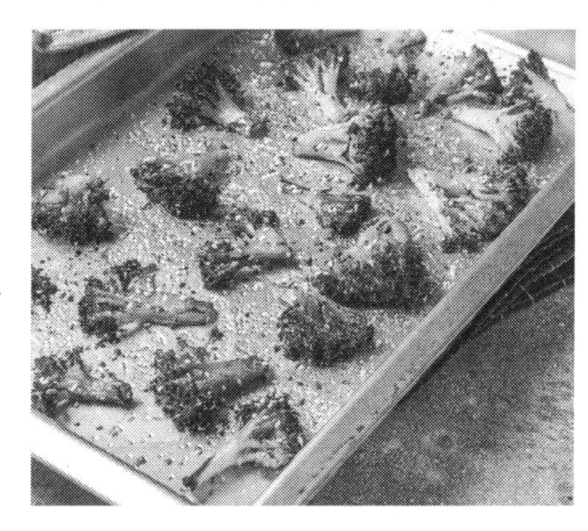

Storage:
Allow to totally cool, then wrap each one in foil or plastic wrap before putting them in an airtight freezer bag and freezing for up to three months..

Reheat:
Broccoli can be thawed in the fridge or heated up from frozen in the oven or microwave

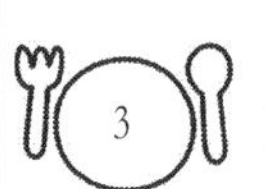  

8.3 Cheesy Squash

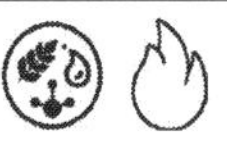 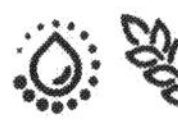 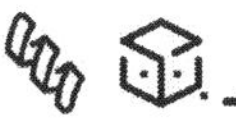 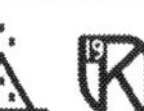

per serving	306 Cal	20.8g	20.8g	12.2g	6.4g	581 mg

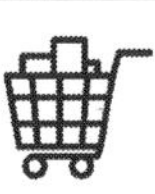

- Salt
- Squash – 2 cups
- Basil , chopped – 1 tbsp.,
- Crumbled feta, 1 1/2 cups
- Olive oil – 1 tbsp.
- Parsley for garnishing

1. Turn the oven's temperature to 425. In a large ovenproof pan (or big baking dish), toss squash with basil, olive oil, and salt.
2. Bake the squash for 20 to 25 minutes, or until it is soft to the fork.
3. When the skillet is done, sprinkle feta over it. The cheese needs another 5 to 10 minutes in the oven to melt.
4. Serve it warm with a parsley garnish.

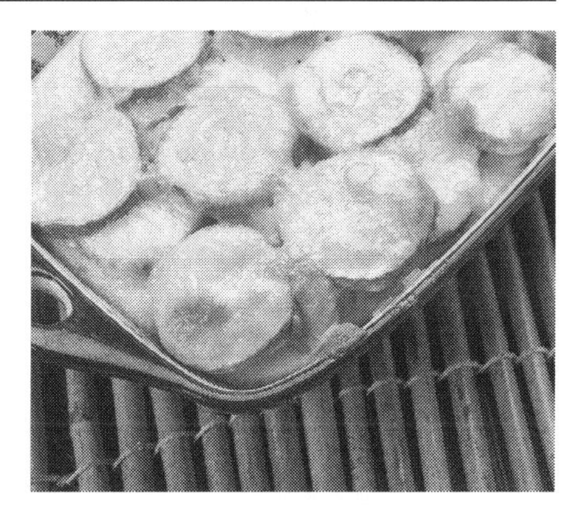

Storage:
Allow to totally cool, then wrap each one in foil or plastic wrap before putting them in an airtight freezer bag and freezing for up to three months.

Reheat:
Heated up from frozen in the oven or microwave

8.4 Grilled Eggplant

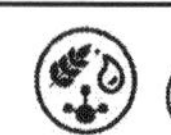 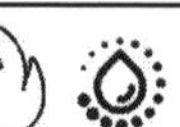 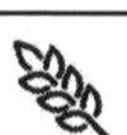 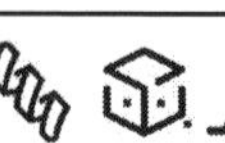 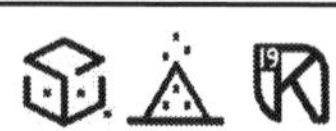

per serving	306 Cal	20.8g	20.8g	12.2g	6.4g	581 mg

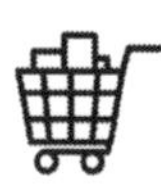

- Dried oregano, 1/2 tsp.
- Salt
- Eggplant, quarter-inch-round slices -1
- 1/2 lemon juice
- Feta crumbles – 6 tbsp.
- Freshly cut parsley, 2 tbsp.
- Olive oil, 1/4 cup

1. Heat a grill or grill pan to high heat before cooking the eggplant. In a small bowl, mix oregano and oil. The eggplants must be lightly dusted with salt.
2. Grill eggplants for two to three minutes on each side, or until they are tender and lightly browned.
3. Before squeezing lemon juice over the grilled eggplants, add feta and parsley.

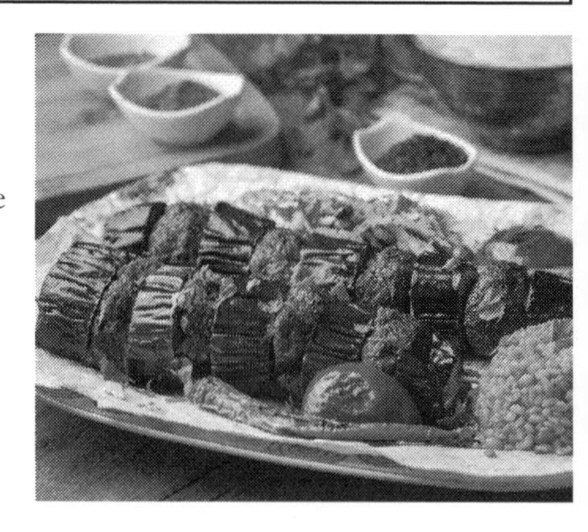

Storage:
Allow to totally cool, then wrap each one in foil or plastic wrap before putting them in an airtight freezer bag and freezing for up to three months.

Reheat:
Heated up from frozen in the oven or microwave

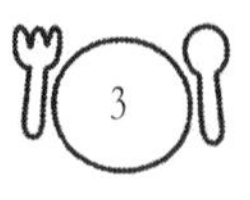  

8.5 Smashed Broccoli

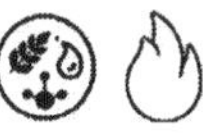 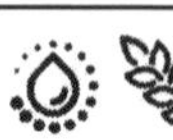 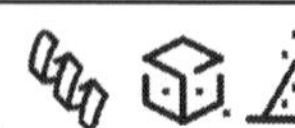 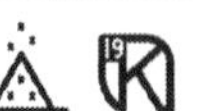

per serving	168 Cal	15.1g	3.4g	6g	2g	100 mg

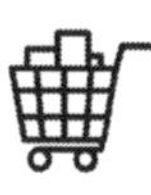

- Lemon juice
- Salt
- Olive oil for cooking
- Half-cup of grated feta
- Broccoli – 1 ½ cups

1. Create a significant ice bath. In a large saucepan of salted boiling water, broccoli should be blanched for two minutes, or until it is bright green and just tender. Drain the broccoli, then immediately place it in an ice bath. The broccoli should be drained once more and dried with paper towels.
2. Just enough olive oil should be added to a large skillet to cover the bottom of the pan. The oil should be heated until it shimmers. broccoli should be added in a uniform layer, and they should be cooked until the bottom of the
3. 3 minutes later, the broccoli is golden and crunchy. Turnover and cook the opposite side until crispy for a further 2 minutes.
4. Broccoli should be taken out of the skillet and placed on a plate lined with paper towels to drain.
5. Immediately sprinkle feta, salt, over broccoli after squeezing lemon juice over it.

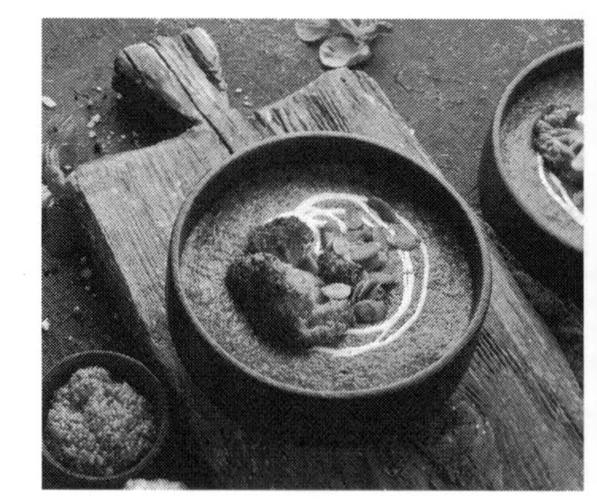

Storage:
Allow to totally cool, then wrap each one in foil or plastic wrap before putting them in an airtight freezer bag and freezing for up to three months.

Reheat:
Heated up from frozen in the oven or microwave

3

12"

21"

8.6 Grilled Green Beans

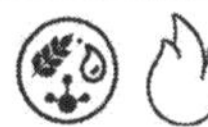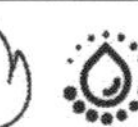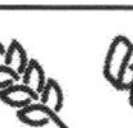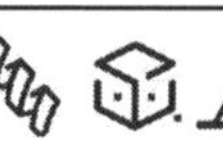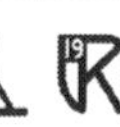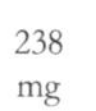

per serving	96 Cal	7.2g	8.1g	2.1g	1.6g	238 mg

- Green beans – ½ pound
- Olive oil, 1.5 tbsp,
- Salt
- Sesame seeds for garnish

1. A big grill pan should be preheated at medium-high heat. Green beans are added and coated after the oil, have been incorporated into a large bowl. Use salt to season.
2. Cook the green beans on the grill pan for about 7 minutes, or until they are completely roasted. (If using a grill, spread a substantial piece of foil over the grates before adding the green beans. Cook as directed.)
3. Sprinkle sesame seeds on top.

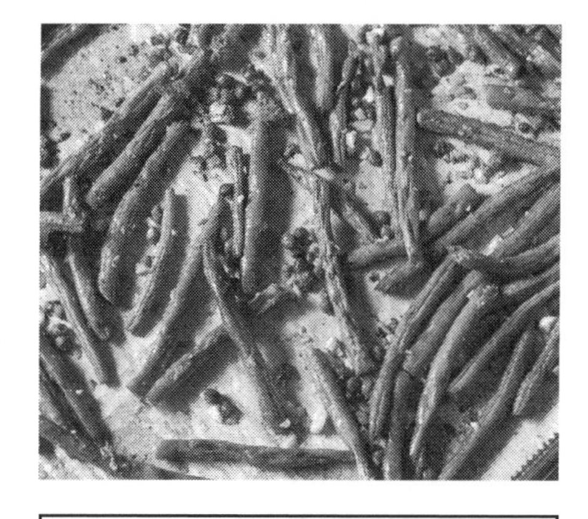

Storage:
Allow to totally cool, then wrap each one in foil or plastic wrap before putting them in an airtight freezer bag and freezing for up to three months.

Reheat:
Heated up from frozen in the oven or microwave

3
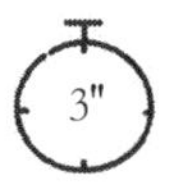
3"

36"

8.7 Easy Roasted Carrots

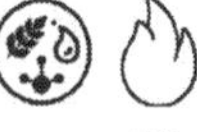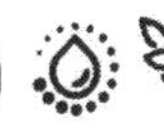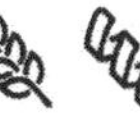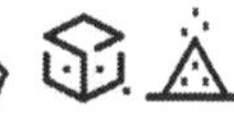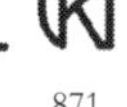

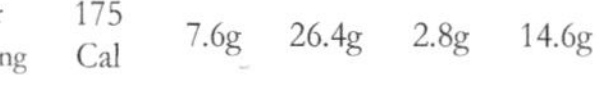

per serving	175 Cal	7.6g	26.4g	2.8g	14.6g	871 mg

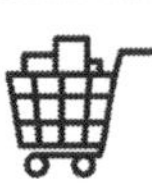

- Carrots, quartered and peeled - 6
- Olive oil - 1.5 tbsp
- Salt
- Parsley, chopped, as a garnish (optional)

1. Set the oven to 400 degrees. On a sizable baking sheet, carrots should be coated in olive oil and liberally salted.
2. Roast for 30 minutes, until soft with a hint of caramelization.
3. Add parsley as a garnish before serving, if preferred.

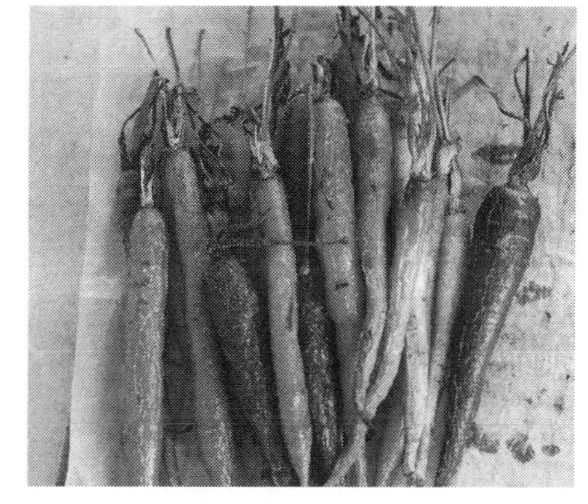

Storage:
Allow to totally cool, then wrap each one in foil or plastic wrap before putting them in an airtight freezer bag and freezing for up to three months.

Reheat:
heated up from frozen in the oven or microwave

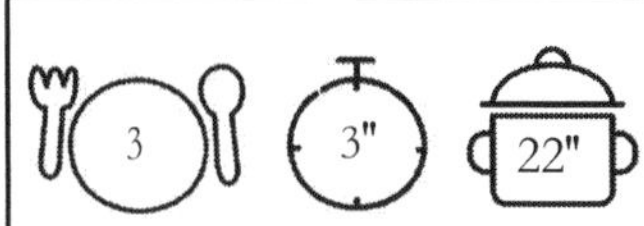

8.8 Sesame Green Beans

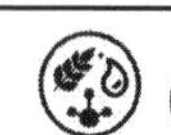 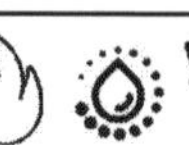 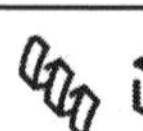 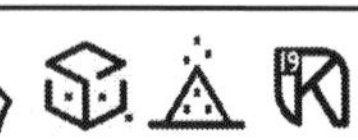 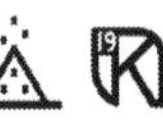

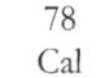 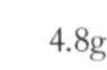

per serving	78 Cal	4.8g	8.6g	2.5g	1.6g	248 mg

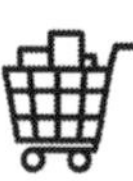

- Olive oil, 1/2 tbsp.
- Sesame seeds – ½ tsp.
- Fresh green beans,– ½ pound
- Water – 1/8 cup
- Salt

1. Over medium heat, warm the oil in a sizable skillet or wok. Include sesame seeds. Green beans should be added as the seeds begin to black. Cook the beans while stirring until they turn bright green.
2. Add water along with salt . For about 10 minutes, boil the beans under cover until they are tender-crisp. Cook without the cover until the liquid evaporates.

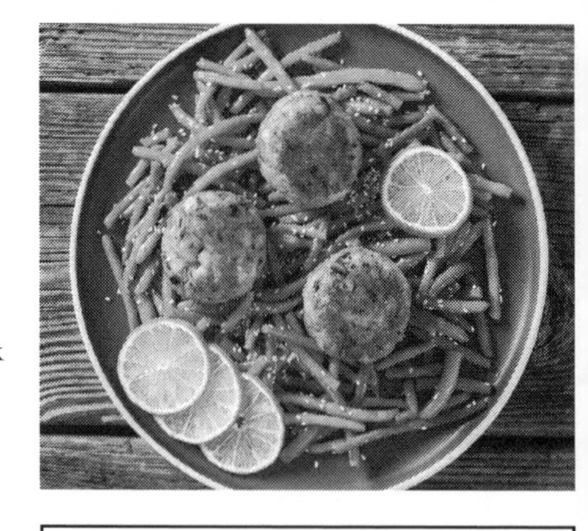

Storage:
Allow to totally cool, then wrap each one in foil or plastic wrap before putting them in an airtight freezer bag and freezing for up to three months.

Reheat:
heated up from frozen in the oven or microwave

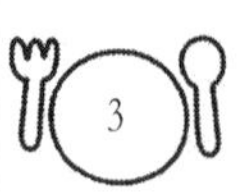  

8.9 Spicy Green Beans

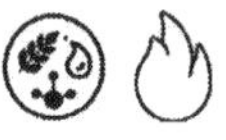  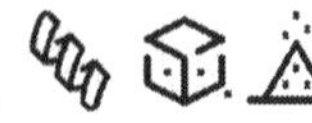 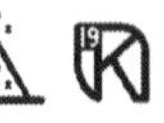

per serving	47 Cal	1.4g	6.1g	1.6g	1.2g	179 mg

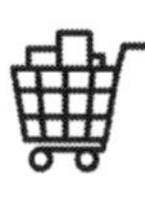

- fresh green beans, 6 ounces, trimmed,
- 1/2 tablespoon garlic infused oil
- 1/2 tsp. apple cider vinegar

1. Add green beans to a dish. A blend of apple cider vinegar and garlic-infused oil should be used to coat green beans. Once coated, toss, and then set aside for five minutes.
2. Place medium-high heat in a stainless steel pot. Cook beans until they start to sweat while covered. Once the cover is off, stir the beans occasionally until they are cooked.

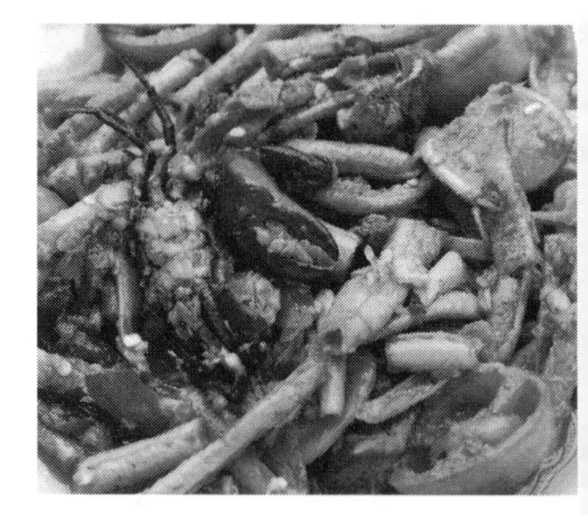

Storage:
Allow to totally cool, then wrap each one in foil or plastic wrap before putting them in an airtight freezer bag and freezing for up to three months.

Reheat:
Heated up from frozen in the oven or microwave

 3 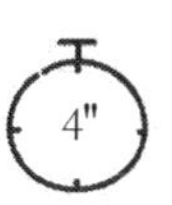 4"  12"

8.10 Lemon-Cilantro Green Beans

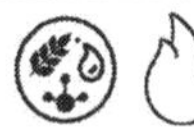 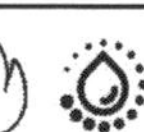 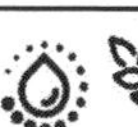 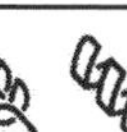 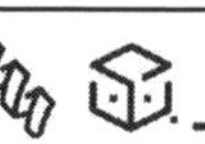 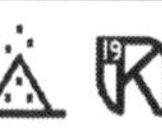 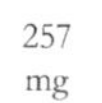

per serving	98 Cal	7.2g	8.8g	2.2g	1.8g	257 mg

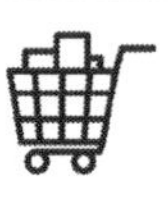

- Cilantro - ¼ cup
- 1 dash of stevia
- Lemon zest - 1 tbsp
- Olive oil-1 tbsp.
- Salt to taste
- Wedges sliced from one lemon
- Fresh green beans, trimmed to 2 cups

1. Over high heat, bring a large saucepan of salted water to a boil. Add stevia and beans. Cook for 3 to 5 minutes, or until beans are brilliant green and soft. To cease cooking, drain the food and place it in a big dish of icy water.
2. Over medium-high heat, add olive oil .Cook the beans for about 4 minutes, stirring occasionally, until the beans are wilted. Add cilantro and lemon zest to the beans and simmer for a further one to two minutes. Use salt to taste to season. Add lemon wedges as a garnish after transferring the beans to a serving dish.

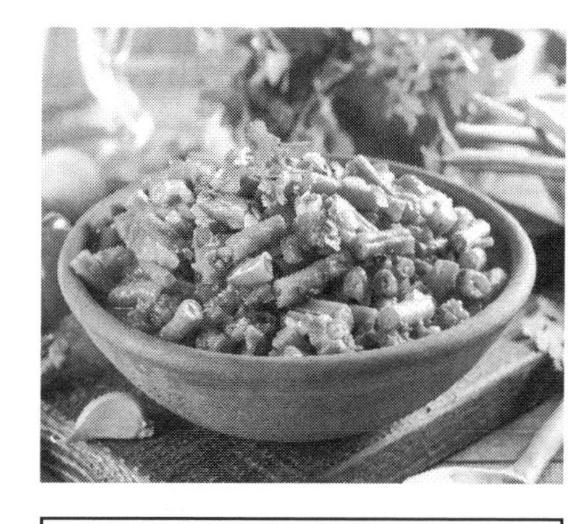

Storage:
Allow to totally cool, then wrap each one in foil or plastic wrap before putting them in an airtight freezer bag and freezing for up to three months.

Reheat:
Heated up from frozen in the oven or microwave

 3  12"  22"

8.11 Lemon Herb Quinoa

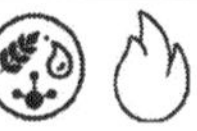 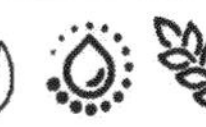 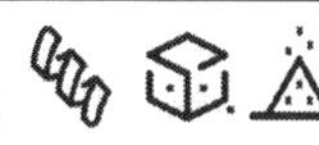 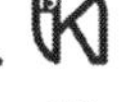

per serving	107 Cal	1.8g	18.8g	4.1g	0.3g	178 mg

- Water, 1 cup
- ½ cup of quinoa
- Lemon – 1 juiced and zested
- Parsley – 6 tbsp.
- Basil - 6 tbsp.
- Salt

1. Place the water, quinoa, lemon juice, lemon zest, parsley, basil, and salt mix in a saucepan. After bringing to a boil, turn down the heat to medium-low, cover the pot, and let the quinoa simmer for 20 minutes, or until the water has been absorbed. Use a fork to fluff after 5 minutes of resting under cover.

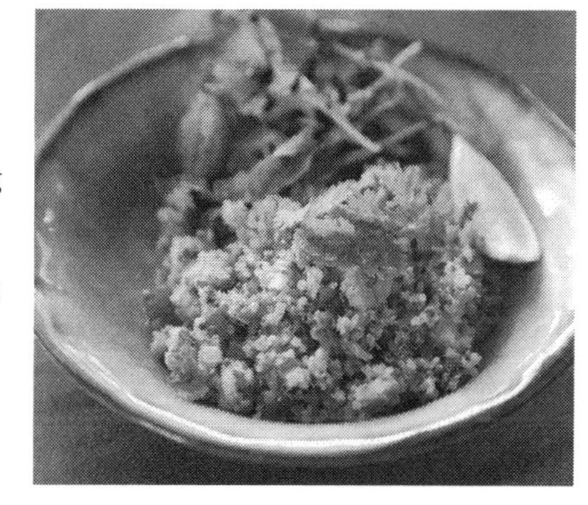

Storage:
Allow to totally cool, then wrap each one in foil or plastic wrap before putting them in an airtight freezer bag and freezing for up to three months.

Reheat:
Heated up from frozen in the oven or microwave

8.12 Kale Quinoa

 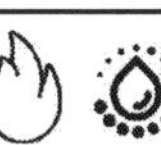 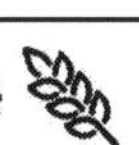 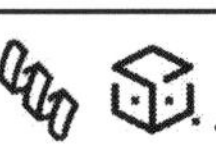 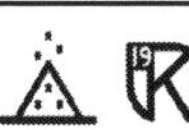

per serving	188 Cal	9.3g	22.2g	5.1g	0g	331 mg

- Salt to taste
- 1 teaspoon of sesame oil
- Olive oil - 1 tbsp.
- Quinoa - 1 cup
- Kale, chopped – 1 cup
- Water - 2 cups

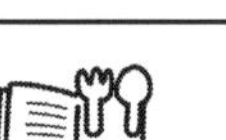

1. Quinoa and cup water are brought to a boil in a pan. Reduce heat to medium-low, cover, and simmer for 15 to 20 minutes, or until quinoa is cooked and water has been absorbed.
2. Bring olive oil to a simmer in a skillet. Kale is sautéed in heated oil for 5 minutes or until kale has wilted. Add salt to taste.
3. As the flavours meld, another five minutes or so, stir in the quinoa and sesame oil mixture. To keep the mixture from sticking, add 1 tablespoon of water.

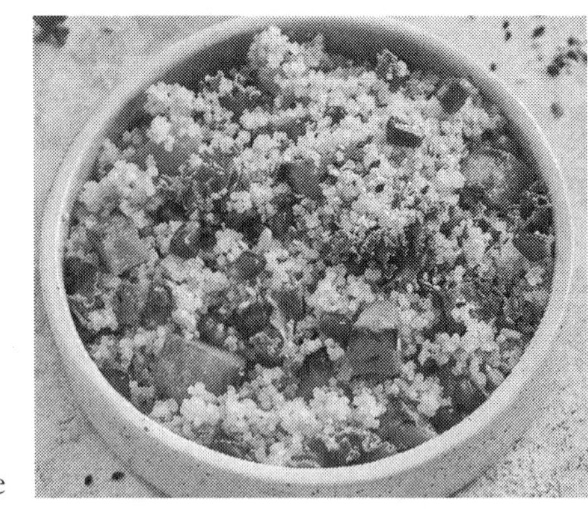

Storage:
Allow to totally cool, then wrap each one in foil or plastic wrap before putting them in an airtight freezer bag and freezing for up to three months.

Reheat:
Heated up from frozen in the oven or microwave

 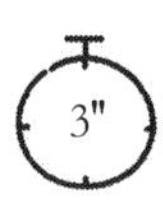 

8.13 Carrot Quinoa

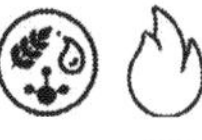 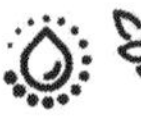 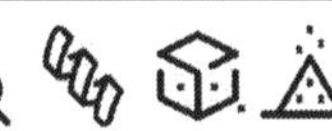 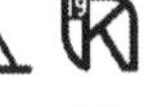

per serving	309 Cal	15.3g	37.8g	7.1g	6g	549 mg

- Green bell pepper – 1
- Carrots – 2
- Water – 2 cups
- Red bell pepper - 1
- Quinoa – 2 cups
- Olive oil, 1/8 cup
- Dried basil

1. Heat the olive oil in a large saucepan over medium-high heat. Carrots, red, green, and green bell peppers should all be included. Cook and stir until softened, about 5 minutes. For about 3 minutes, boil and stir until aromatic.
2. Fill the pot with water and quinoa. Cook the quinoa for about 20 minutes with the lid on. Sprinkle some dried basil on top.

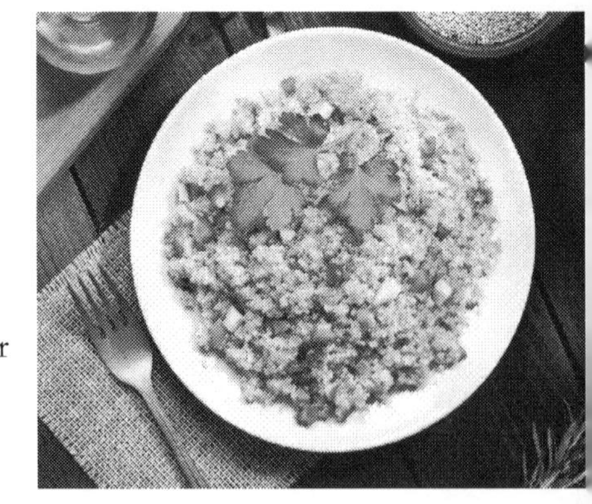

Storage:
Allow to totally cool, then wrap each one in foil or plastic wrap before putting them in an airtight freezer bag and freezing for up to three months.

Reheat:
Heated up from frozen in the oven or microwave

 3  14"  24"

8.14 Olive Oil Roasted Eggplant with Lemon

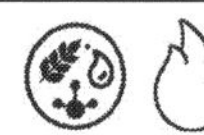 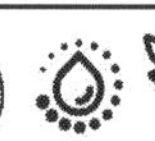 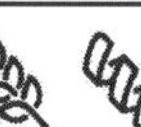 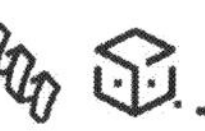 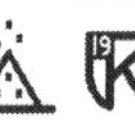

per serving	309 Cal	15.3g	37.8g	7.1g	6g	549 mg

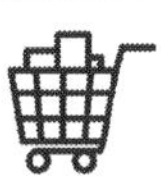

- One huge eggplant
- Salt - to taste
- 2 teaspoons of lemon juice, fresh
- Olive oil, 3 tbsp.

1. Preheat the oven to 400° Fahrenheit (200 degrees C). A baking sheet can be lined with parchment paper or lightly oiled.
2. Divide each side of the eggplant into quarters after cutting it in half lengthwise. Divide each piece in half to form two shorter sections. Place the eggplant skin-side down on the baking sheet that has been prepared. Sprinkle salt and olive oil on the surface.
3. Roast for 25 to 30 minutes in a preheated oven, or until tender and golden brown. Take out of the oven, then top with lemon juice

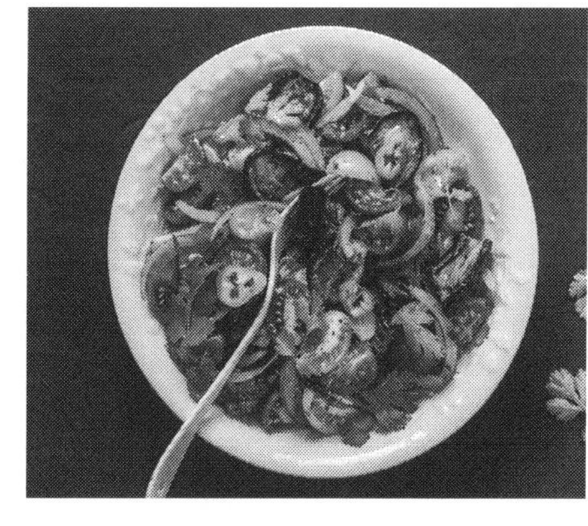

Storage:
Allow to totally cool, then wrap each one in foil or plastic wrap before putting them in an airtight freezer bag and freezing for up to three months

Reheat:
Heated up from frozen in the oven or microwave

 13  14"  6"

8.15 Grilled Eggplant and Zucchini

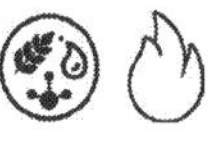 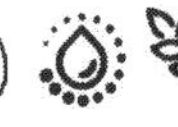 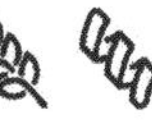 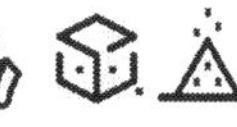 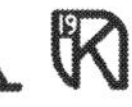 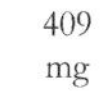

per serving	49 Cal	2.7g	6.1g	1.8g	3.3g	409 mg

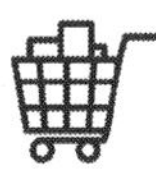

- 6 medium-sized, eggplant, sliced thinly
- 6 zucchini
- 1 tablespoon freshly minced cilantro
- sea salt, one teaspoon
- 20 ml of olive oil

1. Set the oven to 400 degrees Fahrenheit (200 degrees C). Use parchment paper to line a baking sheet or lightly oil it.
2. After cutting the eggplant and zucchini in half lengthwise, divide each half into quarters. Each piece should be divided in half to create two shorter quarters. On the prepared baking sheet, put the eggplant skin-side down. Apply olive oil and salt to the surface.
3. Roast for 25 to 30 minutes in a preheated oven, or until tender and golden brown. Take out of the oven, then top with cilantro. Serve warm.

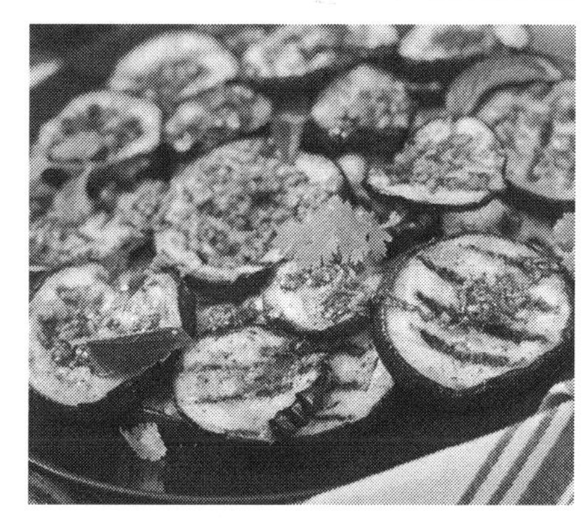

Allow to totally cool, then wrap each one in foil or plastic wrap before putting them in an airtight freezer bag and freezing for up to three months.

Reheat:
heated up from frozen in the oven or microwave

CHAPTER 9

POULTRY RECIPES

9.1 Tandoori Chicken

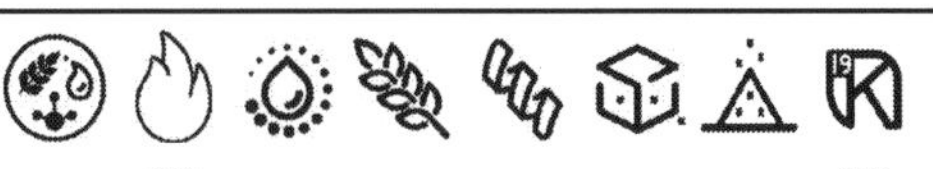

per serving	169 Cal	8.9g	0g	21.1g	0g		178 mg

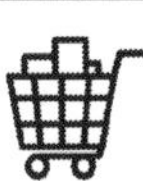

- Coconut yogurt ½ cup
- Tomato puree -2 teaspoon
- Paprika – ½ teaspoon
- Ground Coriander, 1 teaspoon
- 2 teaspoons of salt
- Thick pieces of chicken breast
- Pumpkin 2 cups
- Olive oil – 2 tbsp,.
- Spring onions with thinly cut green tops - 6
- Lime juice – ¼ cup
- Ginger – 2 tbsp,
- Coriander leaves, 3 cups
- To be served: steamed rice

1. By repositioning the oven racks, put one rack in the upper third and another in the lower third. Set the oven's thermostat to 450 F/230 C.
2. Combine the yogurt , tomato puree, paprika, ground coriander, and 2 teaspoons of salt in a sizable mixing dish. Chicken should be added and coated. Allow to rest for at least 10 minutes at room temperature.
3. Place the chicken on a baking sheet with a rim and brush with 1 tablespoon of oil, leaving space between each piece.
4. Mix the pumpkin chunks, 1 Tbsp of oil, and 1 tsp of salt in a bowl. Place the pumpkin on another nonstick baking sheet after coating it.
5. Place the chicken-filled tray on the top oven rack.
6. in the bottom rack. Leave for 15 to 20 minutes to cook. To ensure that the pumpkin cooks all the way through to a tender golden brown, turn it over after 7 minutes.
7. The green tips of 6 spring onions, 1/4 cup fresh lime juice, ginger, 3 cups of coriander leaves, 60 ml of water, 1/4 cup oil, and 2 tsp of salt should be blended until smooth in the meantime.
8. As directed on the rice packaging, steam four servings of rice.
9. Rice should be divided among 3 servings, with chicken, pumpkin, and sauce added on top. Add coriander leaves as a garnish. Enjoy!

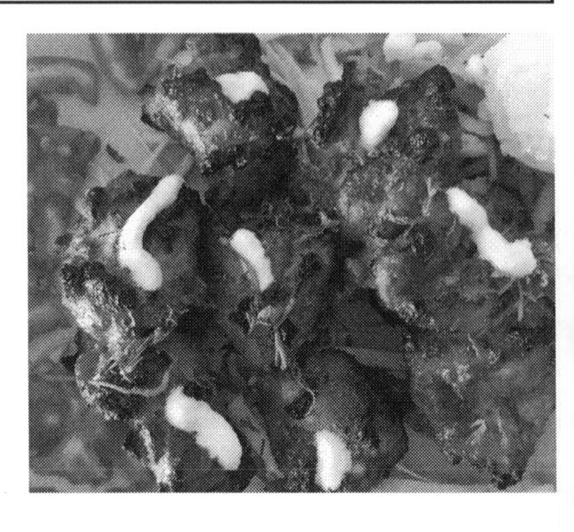

Storage:
For up to 3 days, store in the refrigerator in a tight container. For up to three months

Reheat:
Over medium heat in a large non-stick skillet, warm the chicken by turning occasionally

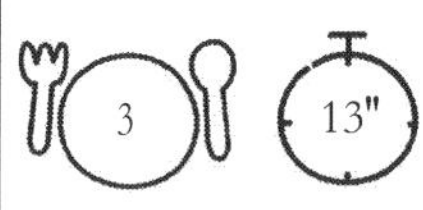

9.2 Lemon Chicken

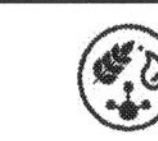 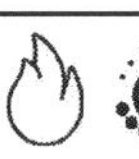 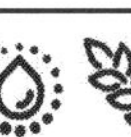 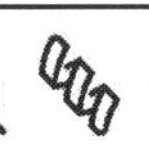 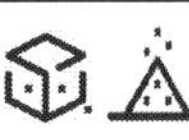 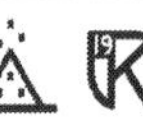

per serving	305 Cal	15.6g	5.7g	36.1g	1.2g	316 mg

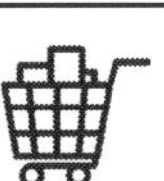

- 1/4 cup almond meal
- Kosher salt, 1 teaspoon
- 1 lemon, divided, into zest and sliced
- Chicken breasts, cut in half, - 2 lb.
- Garlic infused oil – 1 tbsp.
- Parsley, freshly chopped, as a garnish

1. Mix the flour, salt, and lemon zest in a medium bowl. Chicken breasts should be well covered in the flour mixture. The remaining lemon should be thinly sliced.
2. In a large ovenproof skillet, heat the oil over medium-high heat. Adding the chicken breasts in a single layer and cooking them for about 5 minutes, or until the bottoms are browned, is recommended.
3. Cook chicken in a skillet with the water, and lemon slices for three minutes, or until the sauce has slightly reduced.
4. Chicken should be topped with parsley for decoration.

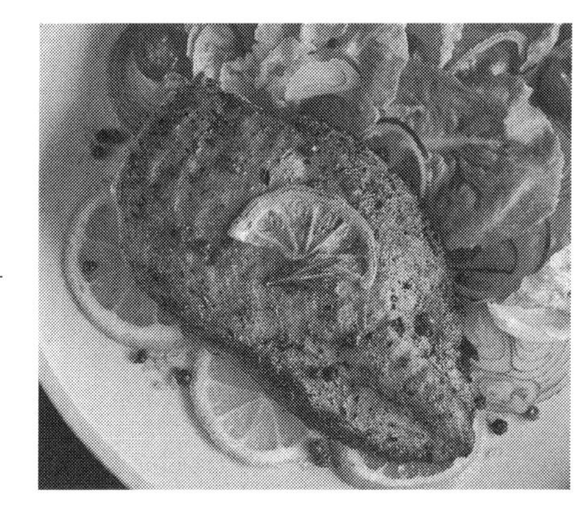

Storage:
The lemon chicken must be individually wrapped and frozen. The lemon chicken should be divided into freezer bags, sealed, and frozen.

Reheat:
Over medium heat in a large non-stick skillet, warm the fajita chicken by turning occasionally.

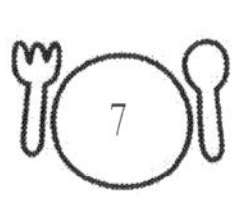

9.3 Cilantro Lemon Chicken

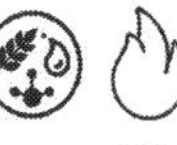 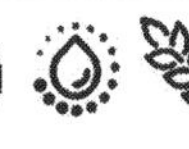 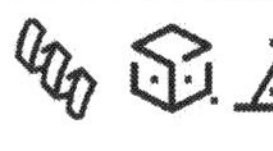 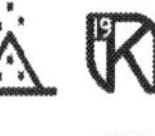

per serving	283 Cal	15.5g	1.8g	32.9g	1.5g	288 mg

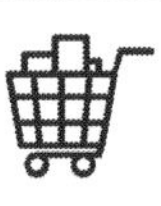

- 1 fresh cilantro bunch
- 1/2 cup of lime juice, fresh
- 4 tbsp, of olive oil infused with garlic
- Olive oil, 4 tbsp,
- 4 tbsp, of stevia
- 1 teaspoon of cumin, ground
- 1 salt
- 3 pounds of skinless, boneless breasts of chicken

1. Combine the cilantro, lime juice, garlic-infused oil, olive oil, stevia, cumin, and salt in a blender. The cilantro should be coarsely chopped after being processed in a food processor.
2. In a container that can be closed, the chicken ought to be near the bottom. To evenly distribute the cilantro lime marinade, turn the chicken. Place in the refrigerator for no more than twenty-four hours, but no less than two.
3. Prepare chicken the way you like it to be cooked: by baking. 450 degrees Fahrenheit should be the oven's temperature setting. Chicken should be taken out of the marinade and put in a roasting tray. After baking for 15 to 18 minutes, insert a food thermometer into the thickest section and take a reading of 165°F. Give yourself five minutes to rest. Slice and serve hot.

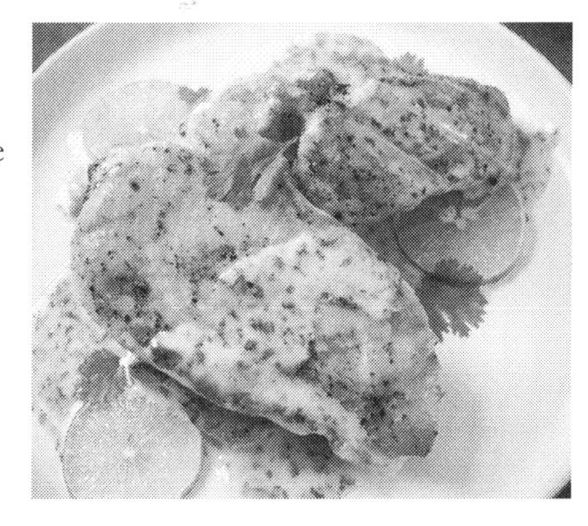

Storage:
For up to 3 days, store in the refrigerator in a tight container. For up to three months, freeze uncooked food in the marinade. Refrigerate frozen foods before cooking..

Reheat:
Over medium heat in a large non-stick skillet, warm the chicken by turning occasionally

 7  12"  24"

9.4 Seasoned Chicken Breast

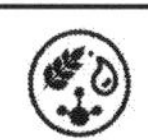 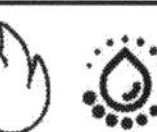 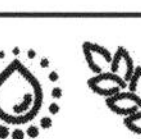 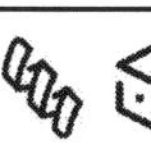 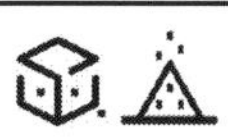 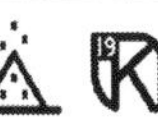

per serving	152 Cal	6.9g	0.8g	20.5g	0.1g		149 mg

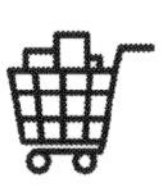

- Cayenne pepper, salt, and pepper to taste
- Breasts of chicken - 7
- Garlic-flavored oil – 3-1/2 tbsp.
- Paprika, 1 tsp.
- Dried rosemary (crushed) - 1-1/2 tsp.
- Mustard powder- ½ tsp
- Dried thyme – ½ tsp.
- Dried parsley – ½ tsp
- Cumin, ground – 1/8 tsp.
- Dried basil – 1-1/2 tsp.

1. Set the oven to 350 degrees. All of the dry ingredients should be completely combined in a mixing dish (or a Ziploc bag).
2. After mixing, chicken is thoroughly covered in olive oil.
3. After removing the chicken from the bowl, place it in an appropriate-sized baking dish (or bag). Bake the dish for 30 minutes with the foil covering. Put the dish back in the oven after removing the foil. Take a temperature reading of the thickest area of the breast every 5 to 10 minutes until it reaches 165 degrees.

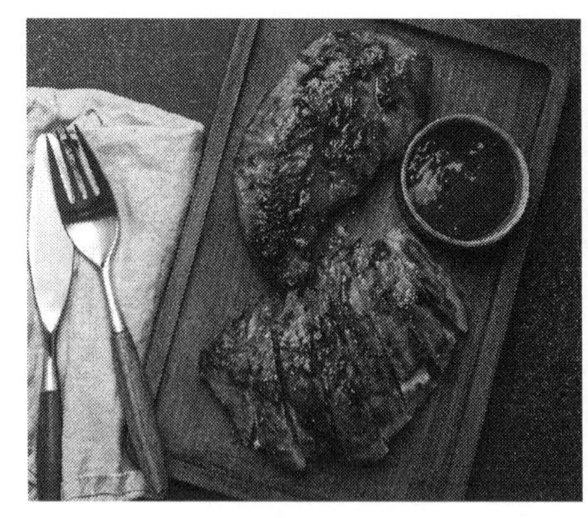

Storage:
For up to 3 days, store in the refrigerator in a tight container. For up to three months

Reheat:
Over medium heat in a large non-stick skillet, warm the chicken by turning occasionally.

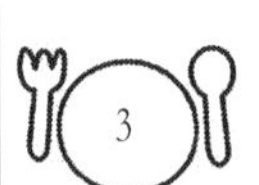 3 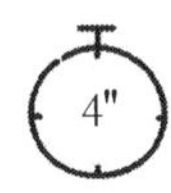 4"  6"

9.5 Chicken Paillard

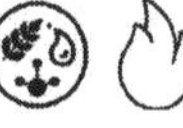  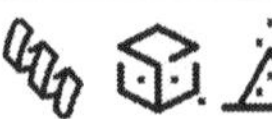 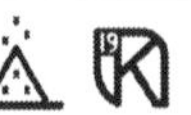

per serving	169 Cal	8.9g	0g	21.8g	0g		178 mg

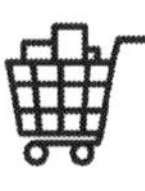

- Two 6 to 8 ounce (170 g to 225 g) skinless, boneless chicken breast halves, at room temperature.
- Salt
- Olive oil

1. Each chicken breast half should have the soft component removed and saved for later use. On your work area, sandwich a breast half between two pieces of plastic wrap. The paillard should be pounded uniformly to a thickness of roughly 14 inches using a flat-sided mallet (6 mm). Instead of tapping the mallet down vertically, move it away from you and softly tap it repeatedly until the chicken is the same thickness all the way around. The other breast half should also be seasoned on both sides with salt and pepper.
2. As a heavy skillet heats up over medium heat, a thin coating of oil should be added to the bottom. You can cook both paillards depending on how big your pan is.
3. You could also prepare each item separately. Do not worry; they cook rapidly. To reduce splatter, place the chicken in the pan with its back to you. Allow to sear, occasionally shaking the pan. Turn the burger over and cook the second side after the bottom has formed a nice crust. The duration shouldn't exceed five minutes. The size and temperature of the breasts will determine this. Serve right away.

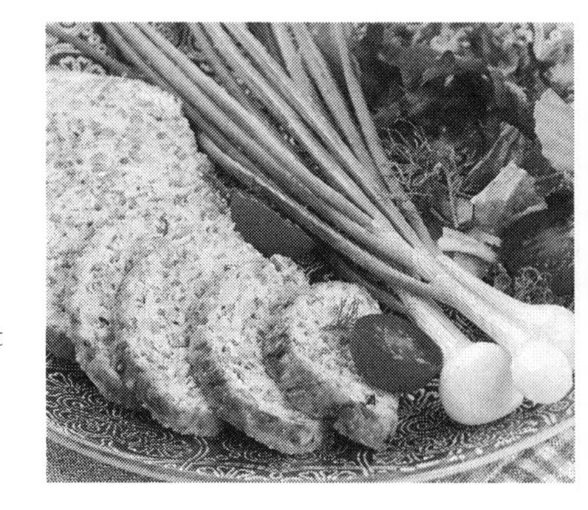

Storage:
For up to 3 days, store in the refrigerator in a tight container. For up to three months.

Reheat:
Over medium heat in a large non-stick skillet, warm the chicken by turning occasionally

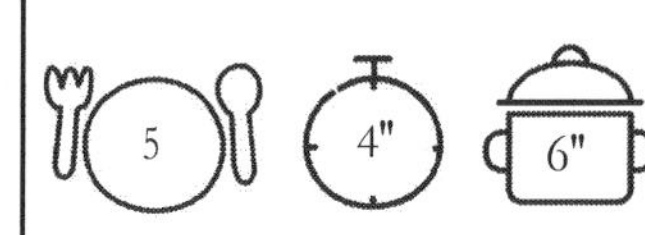

9.6 Chicken Parmesan

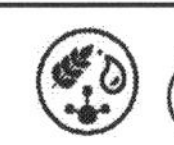 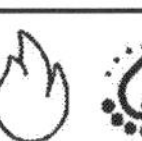 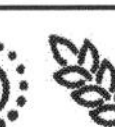 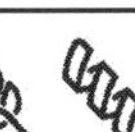 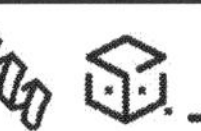 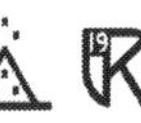

per serving	169 Cal	8.9g	0g	21.1g	0g	178 mg

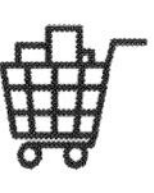

- Olive oil, 4 tbsp,
- Low FODMAP gluten-free spaghetti, or your preferred type of gluten-free pasta, 8 ounces
- Chicken breasts -3 large
- Seasoning mix – 1 teaspoon.
- Beaten egg - 1
- Water – 1 teaspoon.
- Almond flour, half a cup
- 4 ounces or 1 cup of shredded feta cheese
- Fresh basil leaves, cut thinly or whole (optional), 1/4 cup
- Parmesan cheese, 1/4 cup
- Olive oil

1. Following the directions on the package, cook and drain the spaghetti. Season the chicken as desired while the spaghetti is cooking. Add some Seasoning mix on top. In a small bowl, combine the flour and Parmesan cheese. In one more small bowl, whisk together the egg and water.
2. Apply the flour mixture on the chicken first, then the egg mixture, and finally the flour mixture once more. Remove any extra flour mixture by shaking.
3. Heat the oil in a 12-inch skillet over medium-high heat. Cook the chicken for 4 minutes after adding it (making sure that the skillet and pan are hot before adding the chicken to prevent sticking). The chicken should be cooked thoroughly and golden brown after 4 more minutes of turning it over. each chicken piece with a 1/4 cup cheese and 3 tbsp, of sauce. Three minutes should be enough time to melt the cheese under cover. Serve the chicken and hot spaghetti with the remaining sauce. If preferred, top with basil just before serving.

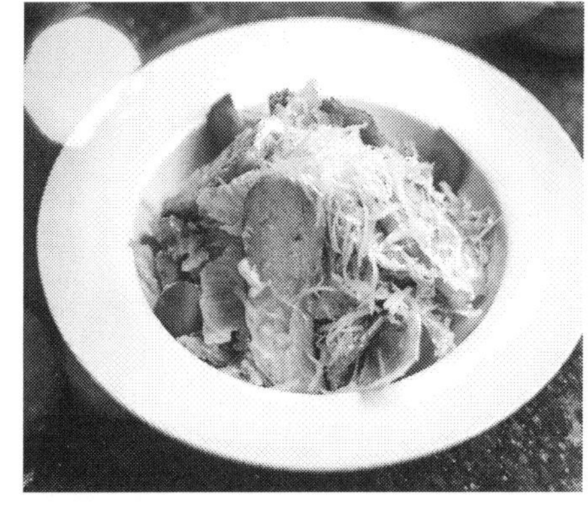

Storage:
For up to 3 days, store in the refrigerator in a tight container. For up to three months

Reheat:
Over medium heat in a large non-stick skillet, warm the chicken by turning occasionally

9.7 Chicken Fajitas

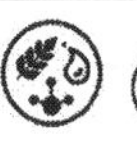  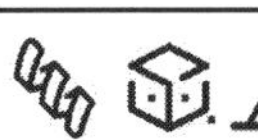 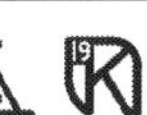 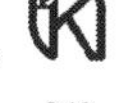

per serving	177 Cal	8g	3.2g	22.1g	2g	260 mg

- Olive oil, - 2 tbsp.
- Lime juice – 1-1/2 cup
- Skinless, boneless chicken breasts – 2 pound
- Salt
- Bell peppers, sliced very thin - 4

1. Mix 1 tbsp. oil, lime juice, in a big basin. Chicken should be salted before being added to the bowl and coated .A minimum of 30 minutes and a maximum of 2 hours should be given for the food to marinade in the fridge.
2. In a skillet, heat the last tbsp. of oil over medium heat when it's time to fry. Cook the chicken, 8 minutes per side, until golden and well done. After 10 minutes of resting, cut into strips.
3. Cook bell peppers in the skillet for five minutes, or until tender. Add the chicken and blend by tossing.

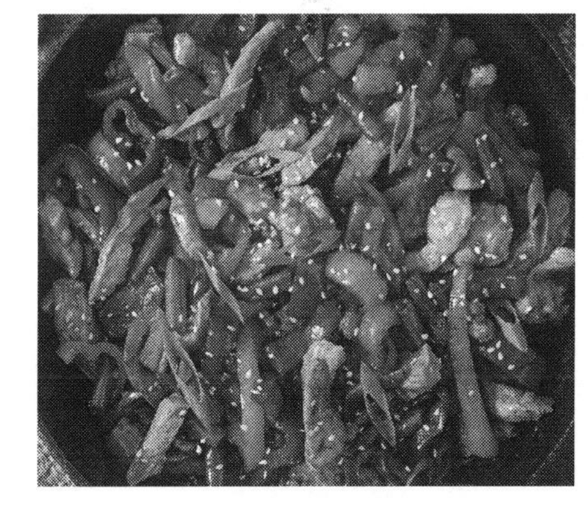

Storage:
The chicken fajita filling must be individually wrapped and frozen. The filling should be divided into freezer bags, sealed, and frozen.

Reheat:
Over medium heat in a large non-stick skillet, warm the fajita chicken by turning occasionally.

 5  11"  39"

9.8 Maple Mustard Baked Chicken

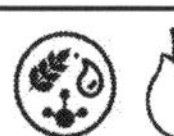 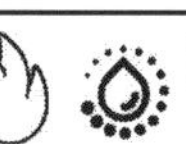 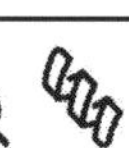 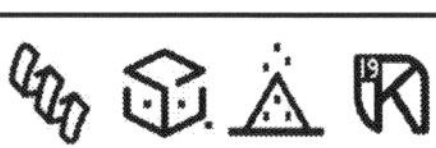 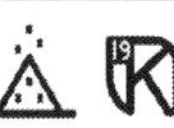

per serving	351 Cal	11.6g	16.3g	41.1g	13.2g		389 mg

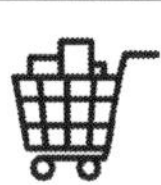

- Ground mustard (or 1 teaspoon dried) – 2 tbsp,
- Maple syrup – 6 tbsp,
- Dried parsley – ½ teaspoon
- Salt – ½ teaspoon
- Dijon mustard, - 2 teaspoons
- Skinless, boneless chicken thighs (chicken breasts work great too) - 1 1/4 pounds of
- Basil, - 1 tablespoon

1. A 350°F oven setting. For easier cleanup, if wanted, line a 13" x 9" baking dish with aluminum foil. Apply olive oil cooking spray on the foil.
2. In a medium bowl, combine the maple syrup, Dijon mustards, basil, parsley, salt. After coating with the maple-mustard mixture, place each chicken thigh on the hot baking pan. The chicken should be covered in any sauce that is left behind.
3. Bake the chicken for 35 to 40 minutes, or until the internal temperature reaches 165 degrees Fahrenheit, in a preheated oven. Serve

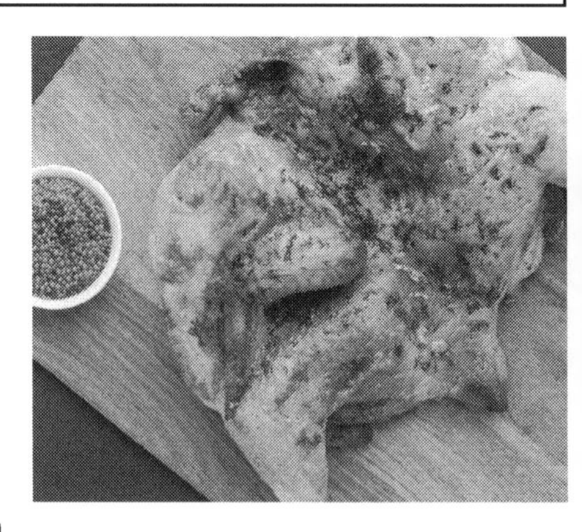

Storage:
For up to 3 days, store in the refrigerator in a tight container. For up to three months.

Reheat:
Over medium heat in a large non-stick skillet, warm the chicken by turning occasionally

 3  11"  9"

9.9 Cajun Chicken

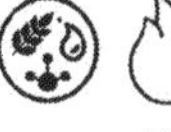  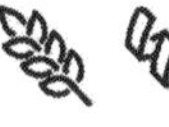 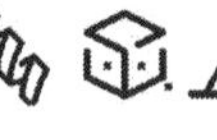 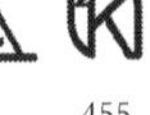
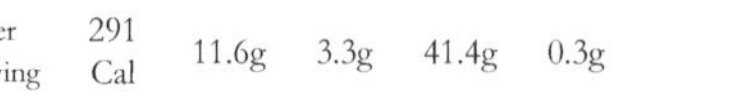

per serving	291 Cal	11.6g	3.3g	41.4g	0.3g		455 mg

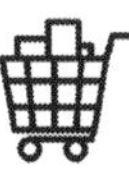

- Chicken breasts - 4
- Sunflower oil – ½ tsp.

Cajun spice blend

- Coriander – 1 tsp.
- Ground cumin,: 5 tsp.
- Black pepper, ground – 2tsp.
- Smoked paprika – 4 tsp.
- Thyme – 4 tsp.
- 1 teaspoon sea salt, flakes
- Cayenne pepper, 1/2 tsp.

1. Make the Cajun spice blend first. Fill a tiny jar with all the herbs and spices, then cover it tightly with the lid. shake well to combine.
2. Each chicken breast should be placed between two sheets of greaseproof paper. Roll the chicken out until it is about 1.5 cm thick.
3. Each chicken breast is spiced with one teaspoon of the spice mixture.
4. Place a nonstick frying pan or grill pan over medium-high heat after lightly oiling it.
5. Cook the chicken breasts for 2 minutes on one side, then flip them over and cook for an additional 2 minutes. Cook the chicken for 1 more minute on each side, or until fully done. There shouldn't be any pink left.
6. The chicken breasts should be placed on a dish to rest for 3–4 minutes.

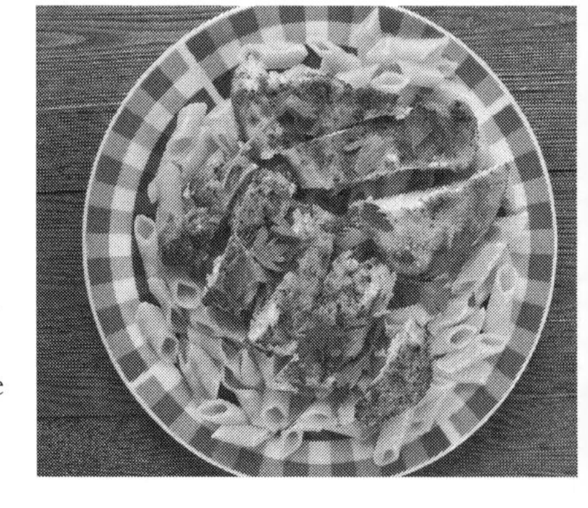

Storage:
For up to 3 days, store in the refrigerator in a tight container. For up to three months.

Reheat:
Over medium heat in a large non-stick skillet, warm the chicken by turning occasionally

 3  11"  19"

9.10 Chicken Dijon

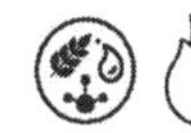  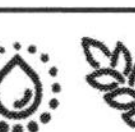 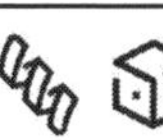 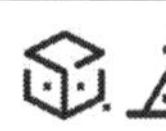 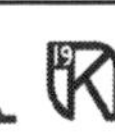

per serving	291 Cal	15.3g	1.1g	33.4g	0.3g	308 mg

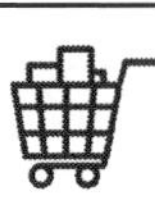

- Salt, 1/2 teaspoon
- White wine vinegar (or Low FODMAP chicken broth) – 4 ml
- Olive oil – 1 tbsp.
- Gluten-free rice flour mixture - 2 tsp.
- ¼ of low-FODMAP chicken stock or broth
- Olive oil, 1 tbsp
- 1 tablespoon of Dijon mustard
- Parsley – 2 tsp.
- Chicken breasts – 16 ounce

1. In a large skillet, preheat the olive oil over medium-high heat. The chicken breasts should be golden brown after 3 minutes of cooking in the skillet. After that, heat should be reduced to medium. The chicken should be cooked for a few more minutes, or until it turns golden brown and reaches an internal temperature of 165 degrees F. To keep warm, the chicken should be moved from the skillet to a dish and wrapped in foil.
2. You can turn off the heat by carefully adding the wine (or chicken stock) and scraping away the browned bits. Re-heat the skillet over a low flame. Add the oil. Blend in the flour. Gradually whisk in the broth. The liquid should be reduced in half while simmering. After that, incorporate the Dijon mustard and parsley. Add salt to taste, if desired.

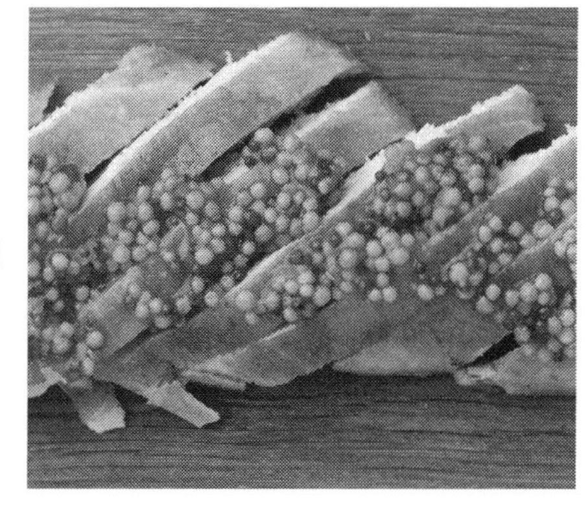

Storage:
For up to 3 days, store in the refrigerator in a tight container. For up to three months

Reheat:
Over medium heat in a large non-stick skillet, warm the chicken by turning occasionally

 3  11"  29"

9.11 Parmesan Herb Chicken

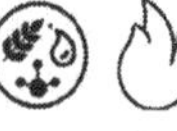 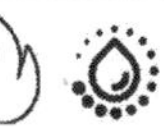 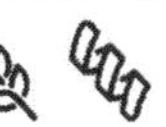 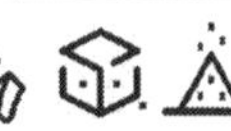 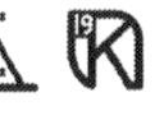

per serving	360 Cal	20.1g	0.8g	42.2g	0g	362 mg

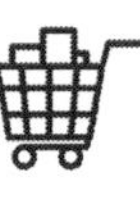

- Grated Parmesan cheese, 2/3cup
- 1 tablespoon freshly minced parsley (or 2 tsp. dried)
- Oregano, dried, two tbsp,
- Salt – ¼ tsp.
- Pepper – ¼ tsp.
- Chicken breast -4
- Olive oil – 3 tbsp.

1. Turn the oven's temperature up to 400 degrees.
2. Combine the first five ingredients in a small plate. Oiled the chicken, then sprinkle the Parmesan mixture on top. Put in a 13" x 9" oiled pan. Spread the remaining cheese and butter on top.
3. Bake uncovered for 25 to 30 minutes, or until the juices run clear.

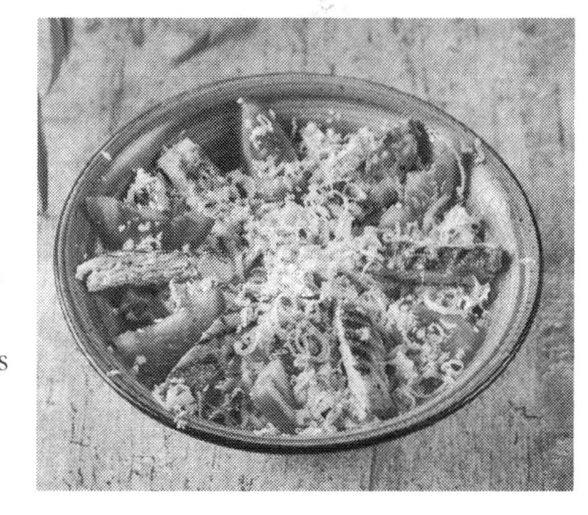

Storage:
For up to 3 days, store in the refrigerator in a tight container. For up to three months.

Reheat:
Over medium heat in a large non-stick skillet, warm the chicken by turning occasionally

5
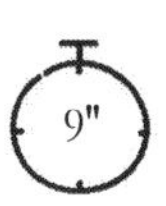
9"

22"

9.12 Lemon Herb Skillet Chicken

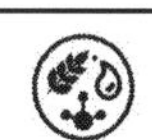 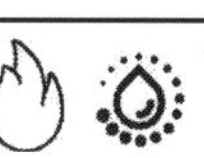 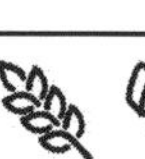 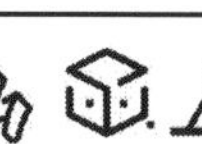 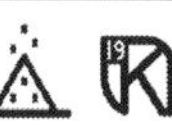

per serving	298 Cal	9.3g	16g	36.4g	0.3g		302 mg

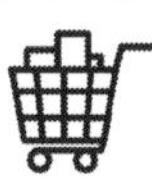

- Chicken breasts – 16 ounce
- Salt
- Garlic-infused oil (or olive oil)- 1 tablespoon
- Low-FODMAP chicken stock or broth – ½ cup
- Italian herbs, 1 teaspoon
- Corn-starch, 1 teaspoon
- Juiced lemon, half (about 1 tablespoon juice)
- Ground black pepper, 1/2 teaspoon
- ½ a lemon, thinly sliced
- White wine vinegar – 6 tbsp,

1. Use a mallet to pound the chicken breast fillets to an equal thickness while they are sandwiched between two sheets of plastic wrap. With salt, pepper, and Italian herbs, season the chicken on both sides.
2. Heat the oil over medium-high heat in a large skillet. Cook the chicken breasts for 3 to 4 minutes on each side, or until browned, after adding them.
3. Put the chicken on a platter, cover the skillet to keep it warm, and turn off the heat.
4. Wine is used to deglaze the pan while stirring to remove any brown pieces. Wine should be simmered in the skillet until it has slightly reduced in volume.
5. Add the chicken stock and cornstarch to the skillet after whisking them together. Add the lemon juice and re-simmer after stirring.
6. Add a slice of lemon to the top of each chicken breast before adding it back to the skillet. Cover skillet and continue cooking chicken breasts until they are no longer pink in the middle or have reached an internal temperature of 165 degrees F.
7. Over rice or noodles, serve the chicken and sauce.

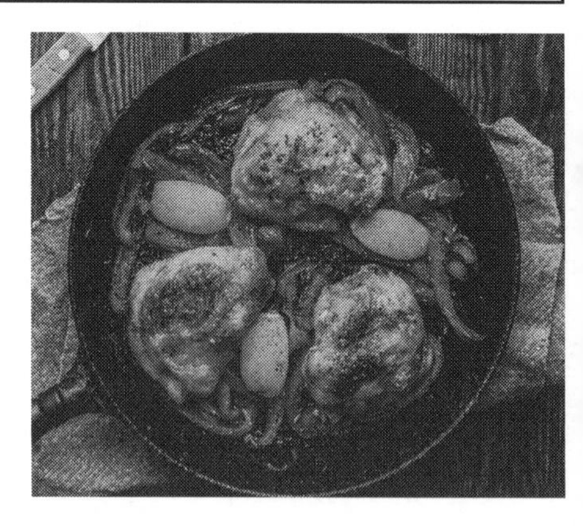

Storage:
For up to 3 days, store in the refrigerator in a tight container. For up to three months.

Reheat:
Over medium heat in a large non-stick skillet, warm the chicken by turning occasionally

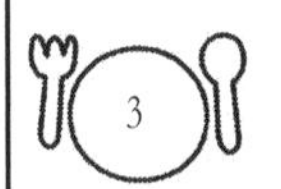
3
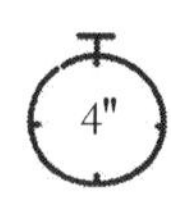
4"

12"

9.13 Sesame Chicken

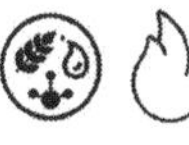 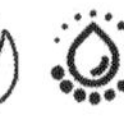 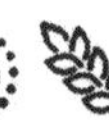 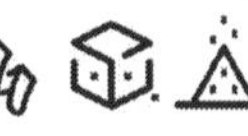 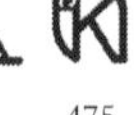

per serving	484 Cal	23g	16.7g	51g	12.8g		475 mg

- All-purpose gluten-free flour mixture – ¼ cup
- Sesame seeds, toasted 2 teaspoons
- 2 teaspoons of crushed black pepper and 1 teaspoon of salt
- 1 and a half pounds of skinless, boneless chicken breasts
- 2 teaspoons of canola oil
- Gluten-free tamari or soy sauce - 6 tbsp
- Sesame oil, toasted 1 teaspoon
- Fresh chives – 6 tbsp
- Brown Sugar, granulated - 1/4 cup

1. The flour mixture, salt, and pepper should be put in a sizable plastic bag that can be sealed. Add the strips of chicken breast and shake vigorously to coat.
2. In a sizable non-stick wok or skillet over medium-high heat, warm the canola oil. Add the chicken and cook it thoroughly for 3 to 4 minutes on each side.
3. Put chicken on a platter, reduce heat to medium, and set aside. Stirring and cooking the soy sauce and sugar in the wok or skillet until the sugar is dissolved. Add the sesame oil and seeds by stirring. Reintroduce the chicken and gently stir to coat. Take the pan off the heat, add the chives, and then serve.

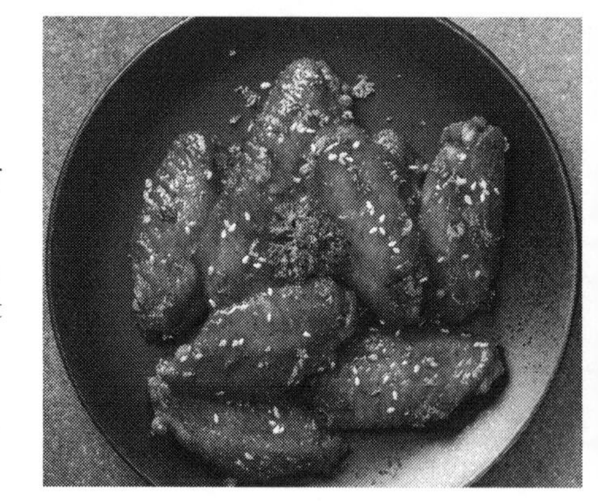

Storage:
For up to 3 days, store in the refrigerator in a tight container. For up to three months.

Reheat:
Over medium heat in a large non-stick skillet, warm the chicken by turning occasionally

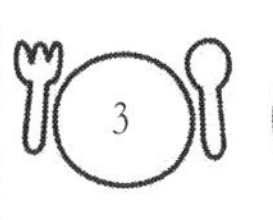 3  9" 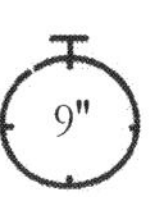 28"

9.14 Chicken Fettuccine Alfredo

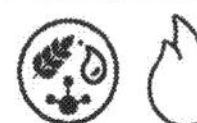 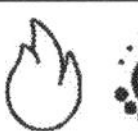 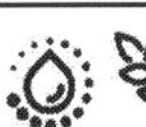 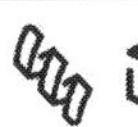 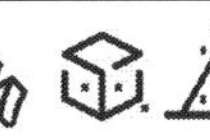 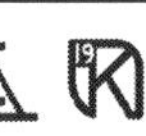

per serving | 363 Cal | 14.8g | 46.7g | 12.6g | 1.1g | 75 mg

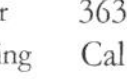 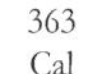 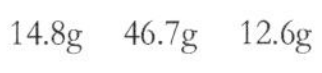 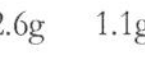

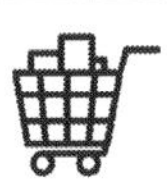

- ¼ cup olive oil
- 8 ounces of gluten-free fettuccine
- 1 - 1 Half a pound of chicken breast tenders
- Ground black pepper, 1/4 teaspoon
- Olive oil, 1 tbsp
- Garlic-Infused Oil, 1 tablespoon
- Shredded Parmesan cheese, 3/4 cup
- 0.5 cups of water
- Chicken Soup Base – 1 teaspoon
- All-purpose gluten-free flour – 2 tbsp.
- Coconut milk, -1 cup
- Freshly cut parsley, 1/4 cup
- 0.5 teaspoons of salt

1. Bring to a boil a sizable pot of water that has been lightly seasoned. After adding it, cook the fettuccine according to the package's instructions. Rinse and drain.
2. While the pasta is cooking, season the chicken tenders with salt and pepper. The olive oil is heated over medium-high heat in a big non-stick skillet. Add the chicken tenders and cook for an additional 3 to 4 minutes, or until browned, on each side. Remove the chicken from the skillet and keep it heated.
3. In a big pot over low heat heat the oil,. Stir in the water and chicken soup base. To remove any lumps, whisk the milk and gluten-free flour together in a small bowl or glass measuring cup. Add gradually while you stir the oil mixture.
4. Continue simmering over medium-low heat, stirring frequently, until the sauce is thick and bubbling. Add the Parmesan cheese and whisk once it has melted and become smooth.
5. Drain and rinse the fettuccine, then toss it with the alfredo sauce. fettuccine needs to be well heated.
6. Arrange the chicken evenly among the four bowls on top of the fettuccine alfredo and garnish with parsley.

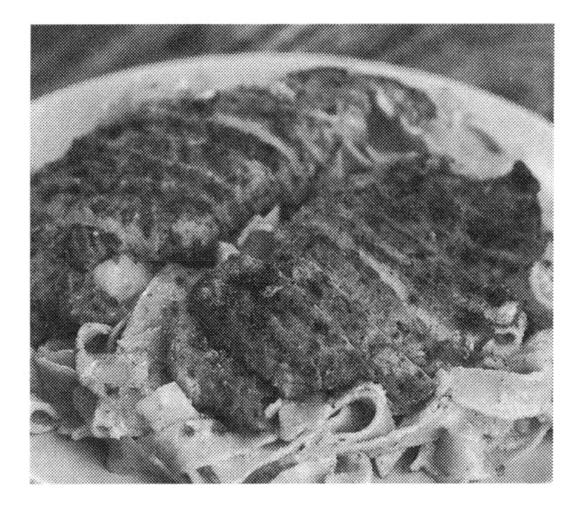

Storage:
For up to 3 days, store in the refrigerator in a tight container. For up to three months

Reheat:
Over medium heat in a large non-stick skillet, warm the chicken by turning occasionally

  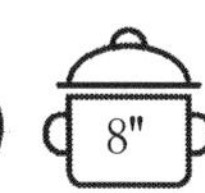

9.15 Greek Grilled Chicken

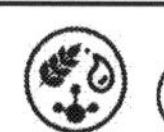 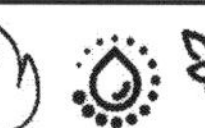 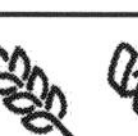 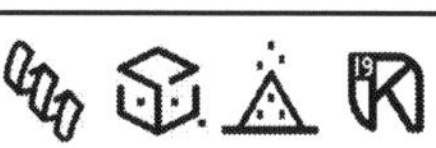 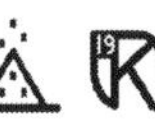

per serving | 283 Cal | 22.2g | 1.2g | 20.5g | 0.2g | 203 mg

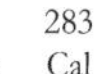 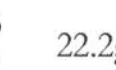 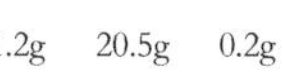 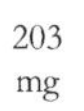

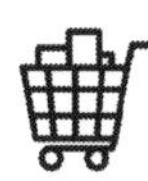

- Lemon juice – 2 tsp.
- 1 teaspoon of oregano, fresh (1 teaspoon dried)
- 14 teaspoon of salt
- 0.5 teaspoons of pepper
- 1 teaspoon of lemon zest, fresh (zest 1 lemon)
- 2, one to one-and-a-half-pound chicken breast halves.
- Garlic Infused Oil,- 1/3 cup

1. To make the marinade, combine the oregano, salt, pepper, garlic-infused oil, lemon juice, and zest in a medium bowl.
2. Half-slices of chicken breasts are used (I usually cut completely through to create 4 thin fillets). Lay each piece flat and pound to a uniform thickness before putting it into a large, sealable plastic bag, one at a time.
3. After placing the chicken breasts in the plastic bag, add the marinade to the entire batch. To coat the chicken, give it a gentle shake. Before sealing the bag, let the air out. In the refrigerator, marinate for a minimum of 30 minutes and a maximum of 2 hours.
4. After lightly oiling the grill, increase the temperature to medium-high (about 350 to 400 degrees F). Chicken breasts should be grilled for 8 to 10 minutes, or until golden.
5. Turning the chicken over halfway through, cook until the internal temperature reaches 165 degrees F.

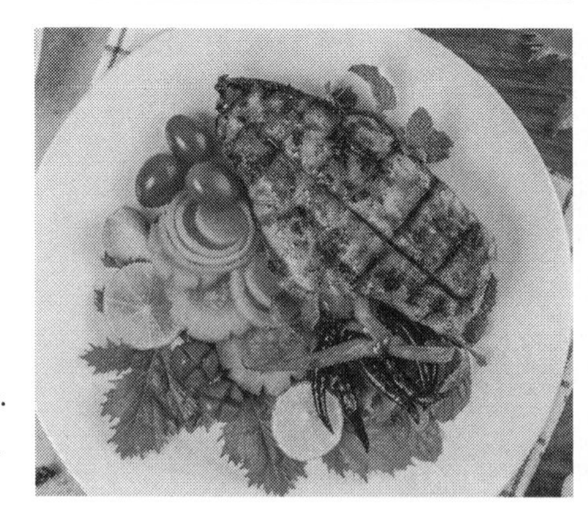

Storage:
For up to 3 days, store in the refrigerator in a tight container. For up to three months

Reheat:
Over medium heat in a large non-stick skillet, warm the chicken by turning occasionally

CHAPTER 10

RED MEAT DISHES

10.1 Beef Tacos

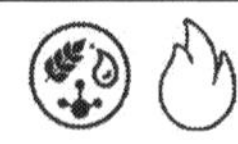
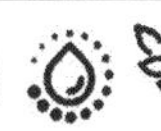
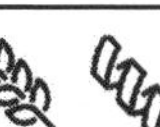
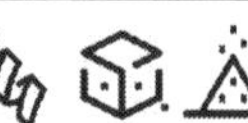
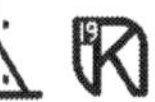

per serving | 241 Cal | 10.5g | 15.2g | 23.5g | 9g | 794 mg

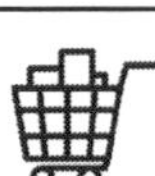

- olive oil infused with garlic- 2 teaspoons
- smoked paprika, 1 teaspoon
- lean beef -1 pound
- Tomato Puree, two tbsp,
- chopped mild green chilies from a 4-ounce can.
- water, 1/4 cup
- cumin, ground -1 teaspoon

For serving,

- Eight tough corn taco shells
- cheddar cheese, shredded- 1 cup
- iceberg or romaine lettuce, finely shred-2 cups
- diced little cherry tomatoes-8

1. Large skillet with garlic-infused oil over medium-high heat. When the mixture is hot, add the ground beef and cook, breaking it up into crumbles, for 5 to 7 minutes, or until browned.
2. In a separate bowl, combine the water, tomato paste, ground cumin, and smoked paprika while the beef is browning. To ensure there are no tomato paste clumps, it takes a little more deliberate mixing, but it saves a meal.
3. Add the tomato mixture and the green chilies in a can once the beef has finished cooking. Cook everything for a further 2 to 3 minutes, or until it is heated. Get rid of the heat. Add salt and pepper to taste.
4. Serve taco beef warm in taco shells made of firm corn. Add up to 2 tbsp, of shredded cheddar cheese, 1/4 cup of shredded lettuce, and 1 diced cherry tomato on the top of each taco.

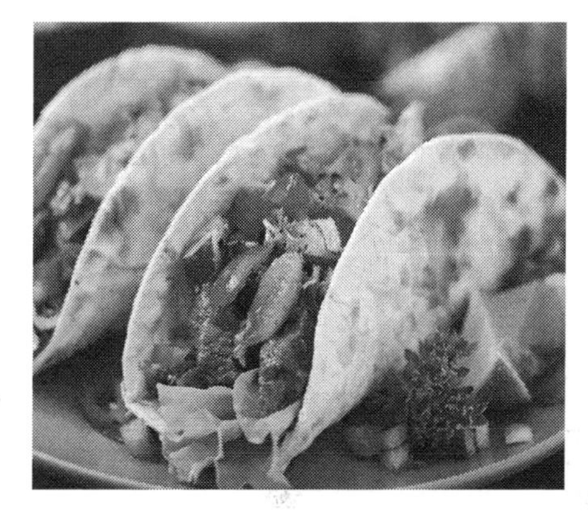

Storage:
For three to four days, the cooked taco meat can be kept separately in the refrigerator in an airtight container.

Reheat:
Empty the filling into a bowl that can be heated in the microwave, then place a tortilla on top of the paper towel you used to cover the bowl. When I put the taco back together, it tasted so good.

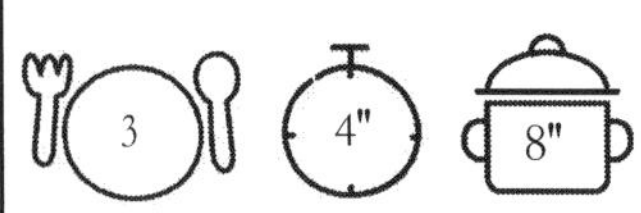

10.2 Quick Korean Beef

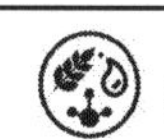 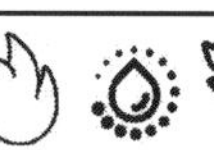 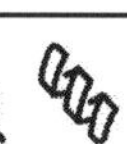 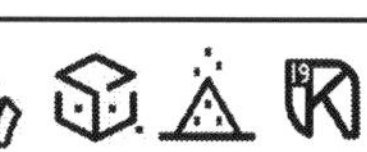 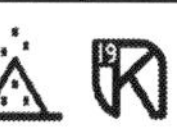

per serving	259 Cal	11.7g	1.6g	35.5g	1.2g	478 mg

- 2Sodium-free soy sauce – ¼ cup
- Finely ground ginger- ½ teaspoon
- ½ teaspoon of red pepper flakes
- Garlic-infused oil-1 tablespoon
- Lean beef - 1 lb.
- Toasted sesame oil - 2 tbsp
- Chopped scallions, only the green bits -1/4 cup
- Optional white sesame seeds-1/4 cup
- Firmly packed 1/4 cup light brown sugar

1. In a small bowl, stir together the ginger, red pepper flakes, brown sugar, soy sauce, and toasted sesame oil.
2. Your wok or a sizable, deep skillet should be heated over medium-high heat. When the oil is shimmering, add it. Hand-crack the meat before adding it to a hot pan or wok. Stir-fry the beef, breaking it up as you go with a spatula. Add the sauce after a minute or two, or when the beef is around halfway done cooking, and stir-fry for an additional minute or two, or until the steak is thoroughly cooked. Give the beef one last toss before including the scallions and sesame seeds, if using.
3. Serve right away with warm white or brown rice.

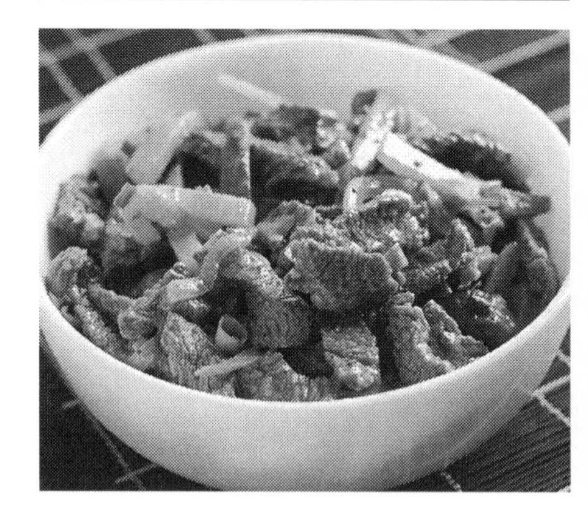

Storage:
Up to 3 days if they are stored in an airtight container in the refrigerator. (By the way, this is a fantastic lunch to bring to work.)

Reheat:
Reheating leftovers in the microwave or on the stove top .

 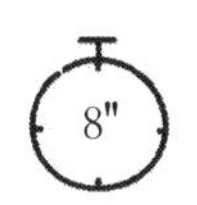 

10.3 Beef Stroganoff

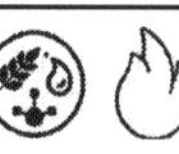 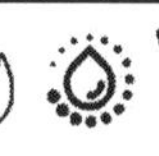 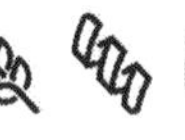 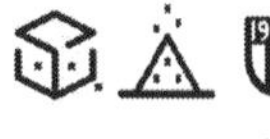 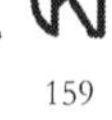

per serving	406 Cal	27.4g	12.6g	26.1g	3.8g	159 mg

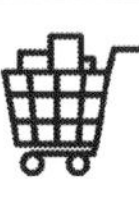

- Rib eye steak, 300 grams, finely split into strips
- butter,- 3 tbsp
- garlic-infused oil, 2 tbsp.
- chopped spring onions (only the green parts)-4
- gluten-free flour -2 Tbsp.
- Low FODMAP beef broth- 500 ml
- Dijon mustard- 150 g.
- Sour Cream without lactose,- 2/3 cup
- salt, and pepper

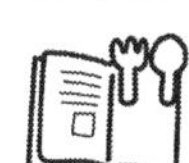

1. Place a Dutch oven or other sizable deep pan over high heat. When the oil is hot enough, add 2 tbsp of beef strips in a single layer and cook for 1 minute on each side without stirring. Cook until just browned and the color is gone. If necessary, sear the steak in two batches to prevent crowding the pan. Put the meat on a plate, cover it, and keep it warm.
2. Add 2 tbsp, of butter, chopped spring onions. Spring onion should be sautéed for 6 to 8 minutes, or until liquid has evaporated and they are tender and gently browned.
3. Stirring continuously, add 2 Tbsp of flour and Sautee for 1 minute.
4. Stir in the first half of the broth. Add remaining broth after it has been combined.
5. Add sour cream and Dijon mustard after stirring. Don't worry if it looks split; the sour cream will "melt" as it heated as you stir.
6. heat to a simmer before lowering to a medium-low setting. Salt and pepper should be adjusted to taste once it has thickened to the consistency of pouring cream (3 to 5 minutes).
7. Add more meat (including plate juices). After one minute of simmering, remove from stove.
8. Serve with rice, quinoa, pasta, or mashed potatoes.

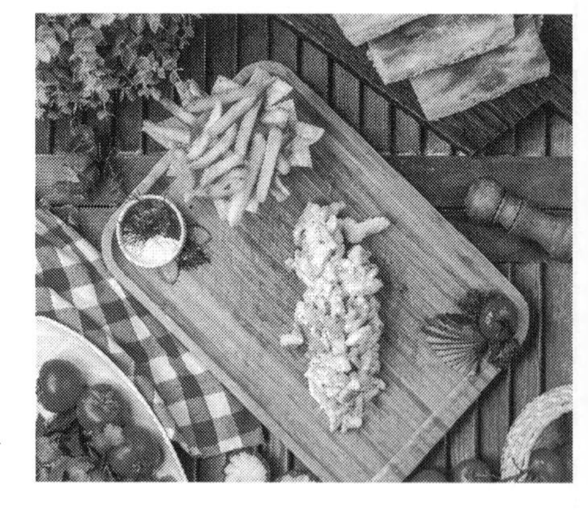

Storage:
Up to 3 days if they are stored in an airtight container in the refrigerator. (By the way, this is a fantastic lunch to bring to work.)

Reheat:
Reheating leftovers in the microwave or on the stove top .

 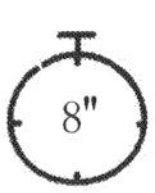 

10.4 Beef Turmeric Rice

 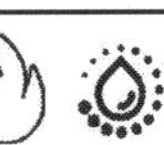 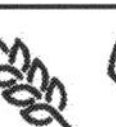 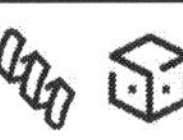 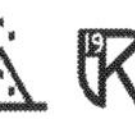

per serving	368 Cal	19.4g	21g	11.4g	3.8g	418 mg

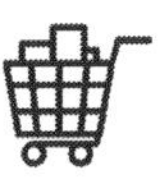

- garlic-infused oil OR olive oil -3 tbsp,
- beef steak- 3 tbsp, of
- Turmeric -1 Tbsp
- medium-grain white rice -1 cup
- big carrot, cut finely- 1 cup
- sea salt,
- canned chickpeas -1/2 cup

1. In a sizable non-stick frying pan, heat the olive oil over medium-high heat.
2. Add the beef and turmeric to the pan, tossing frequently to promote equal browning, and cook for 2 to 3 minutes, or until golden.
3. With the lid on, simmer the beef for roughly 20 minutes at medium heat, stirring regularly.
4. Rice, carrots, and chickpeas should now be added. Recover with water. Bring to a boil, season with salt, and then turn down the heat. Once all the water has been absorbed and the rice is cooked, simmer covered for an additional 15 minutes. Give everything a thorough toss and add more salt and pepper if desired.
5. Remove from the heat and let stand for a further 15 minutes covered.

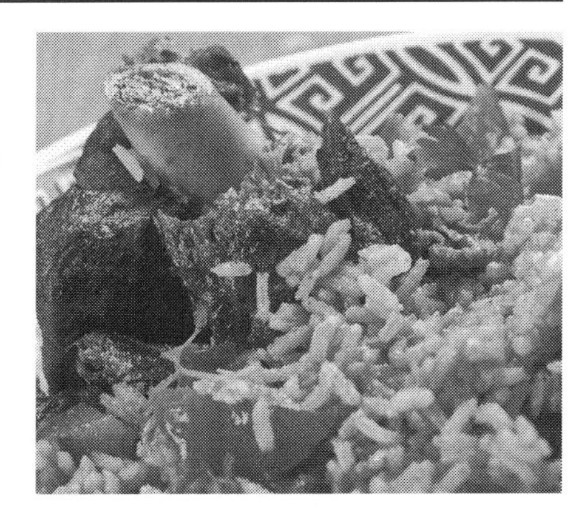

Storage:
Up to 3 days if they are stored in an airtight container in the refrigerator. (By the way, this is a fantastic lunch to bring to work.)

Reheat:
Reheating leftovers in the microwave or on the stove top .

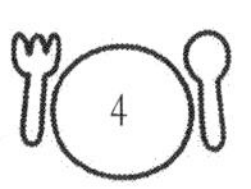  

10.5 Beef Meatballs

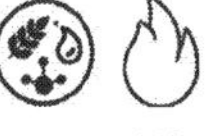 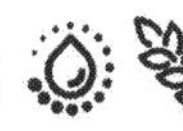 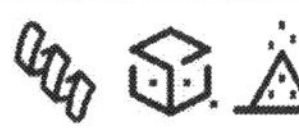 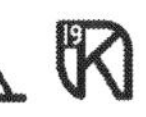

per serving	142 Cal	4.8g	2.4g	20g	0.8g	276 mg

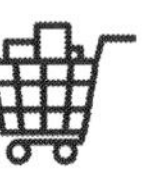

- Pork, ground -250 g
- beef, ground -250 g
- bread free of gluten -3 pieces
- salt, and pepper to taste
- Eggs -2
- grated parmesan -100 gram
- Italian herb blend, 2 teaspoons
- Olive oil with garlic flavouring,- 3 tbsp,
- lightweight frying oil

1. Slices of bread should be briefly submerged in water to achieve total softening. Add them to a sizable mixing bowl after draining.
2. Then, add the remaining ingredients to the bowl and thoroughly blend everything.
3. Heat up cooking oil in a pan if you plan to fry. Add the formed meatballs to the hot oil to begin frying them. Fry till golden brown, turning frequently.
4. Set the oven to 200C if you plan to bake. Place the meatballs on a baking sheet covered with parchment paper. Bake the meatballs for 25 to 30 minutes, or until the outsides are crisp and golden brown.
5. Include the cooked meatballs in the marinara sauce.
6. Serve with quinoa pasta over spaghetti.

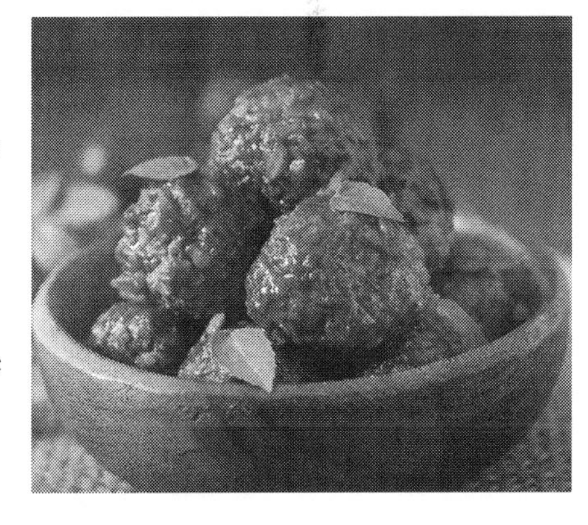

Storage:
Up to 3 days if they are stored in an airtight container in the refrigerator. (By the way, this is a fantastic lunch to bring to work.)

Reheat:
Reheating leftovers in the microwave or on the stove top .

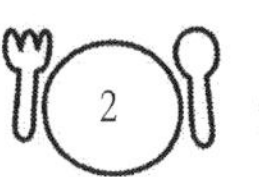
2
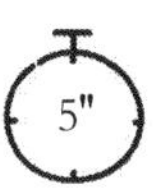
5"

10"

10.6 Spanish Beef and Rice Casserole

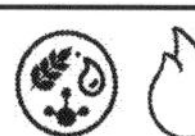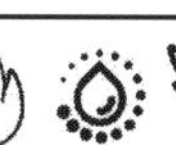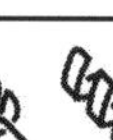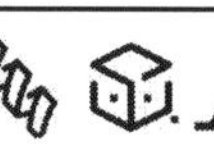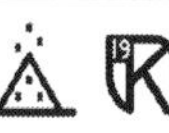

per serving | 467 Cal | 17.8g | 31.5g | 44.5g | 1.8g | 624 mg

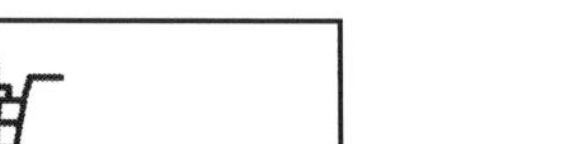

- Water -1.5 cups
- Chopped scallions, only the green parts (about 1 bunch) -1 cup
- 1 lb. lean ground beef
- Long-grained white rice -6 ounces
- Green bell pepper, chopped -1/4 cup
- 1 cup of vinegar
- 1 teaspoon of salt
- 1 teaspoon of brown sugar
- Cumin powder - 1/8 teaspoon
- Ancho chili pepper, half a teaspoon (or as tolerated)
- Black pepper, ground -1/8 teaspoon
- Cheddar cheese, shredded-1 cup
- For garnish, freshly cut cilantro
- Undrained, unsalted diced tomatoes -1-1/2 cups

1. Over medium-high heat, brown and crumble the beef in a big skillet. Remove fat.
2. Stir the remaining ingredients into the beef in the skillet (except for the cheese and cilantro). Heat to a rolling boil over medium-high. Reduce heat to low and slowly simmer, covered, for about 30 minutes, stirring occasionally, until the majority of the liquid is absorbed.
3. Oven temperature set at 375 F. The mixture should be put into a 2.5 qt. casserole dish. Sprinkle cheese evenly. Bake the casserole for 10 to 15 minutes, or until it is hot and bubbling and the cheese has melted. If preferred, garnish with cilantro before serving.

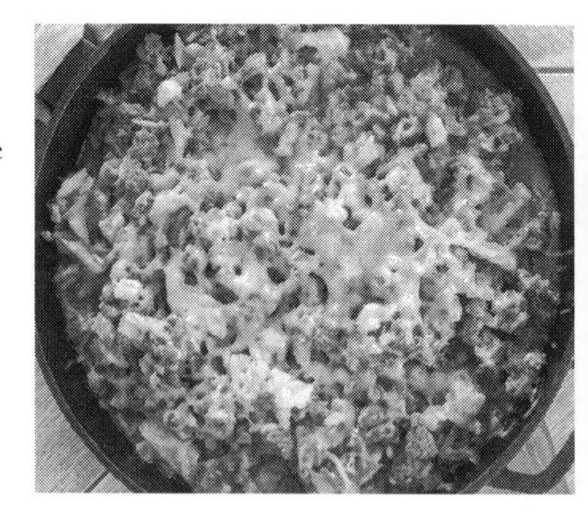

Storage:
Up to 3 days if they are stored in an airtight container in the refrigerator. (By the way, this is a fantastic lunch to bring to work.)

Reheat:
Reheating leftovers in the microwave or on the stove top

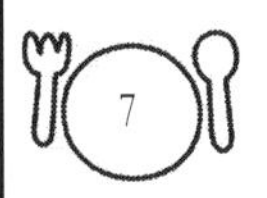
7

8"

42"

10.7 Meatloaf

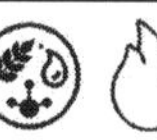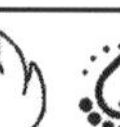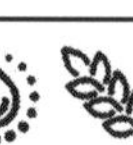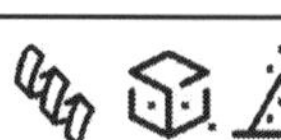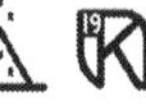

per serving | 167 Cal | 6.8g | 0.5g | 25.1g | 0.1g | 390 mg

- Freshly chopped oregano -2 tbsp. or dried oregano -1/2 tsp.
- Dried chives, 1 teaspoon
- Unbroken egg -1
- Salt -3/4 teaspoon
- Poultry Seasoning, -2 tsp
- Fresh chopped basil -1 tbsp.
- ¼ cup of maple chipotle ketchup
- Ground pork – 1 lb.
- Grass-fed beef – 1 lb.

1. Set your oven's temperature to 400 degrees. Mix the remaining ingredients thoroughly with the ground beef in a large bowl.
2. Place the entire mixture in a 9 x 5 loaf pan and press down to distribute it evenly. For more uniform baking, press down a little harder in the center.
3. Bake in the preheated oven for roughly 45 minutes, or until the center is barely no longer pink. Avoid overcooking by making a tiny cut just in the middle.
4. Before slicing and serving, let sit for 5 minutes. You may also serve with potatoes on the side or over cooked greens, or both!

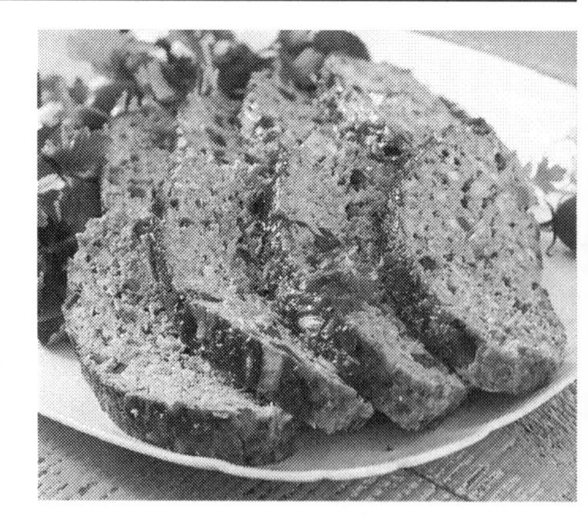

Storage:
Up to 3 days if they are stored in an airtight container in the refrigerator. (By the way, this is a fantastic lunch to bring to work.)

Reheat:
Reheating leftovers in the microwave or on the stove top

5 | 13" | 14"

10.8 Vegetable and Ground Beef Skillet

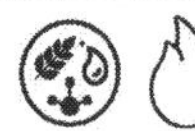 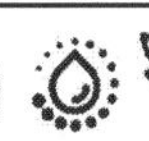 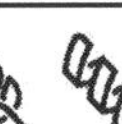 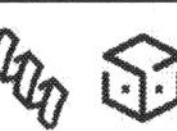 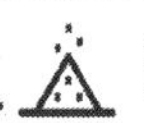 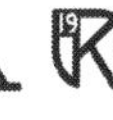

per serving	288 Cal	14.8g	12.5g	26.1g	5g		611 mg

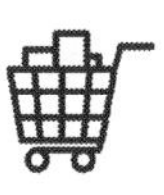

- Olive oil or avocado oil -1 tablespoon
- Big, peeled, and chopped carrots -2
- Radishes -6
- Large crown broccoli, chopped -1
- Ground beef from grass-fed cows, 1 lb.
- To taste, 1 teaspoon sea salt
- Ground ginger -2 teaspoons optional
- Medium zucchini -2 sliced
- Yellow squash, cut -1

1. Large (12-inch) cast iron skillet with avocado oil over medium heat. Stir well after including the radishes, broccoli, and carrots. For about 5 minutes, with the lid on, simmer the vegetables while tossing occasionally.
2. Place the ground beef in the cast iron skillet and push the vegetables to one side. Make a layer of meat by pressing the beef against the skillet. Ginger powder and sea salt should be added. Give the steak two minutes to brown before turning it over and giving it another two minutes to finish browning. With a spatula, shred the steak into small pieces, then toss it into the vegetables to thoroughly incorporate them.
3. Add the zucchini and yellow squash, then cover. Cook for about 5 minutes, stirring regularly, or until beef is well cooked and vegetables are cooked to your preference. As desired, add sea salt to the veggie and ground meat skillet to taste.

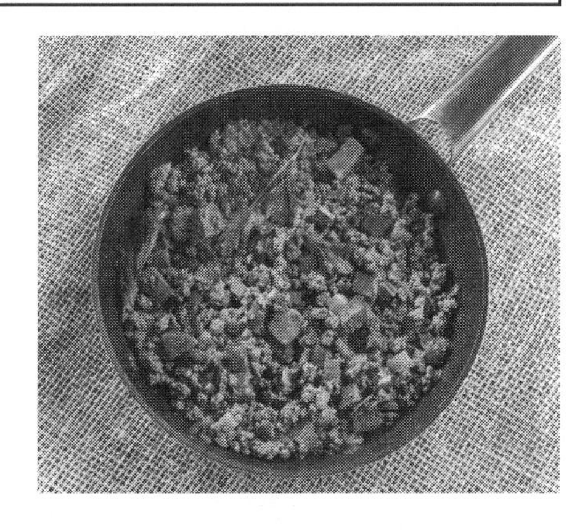

Storage:
is possible for up to 3 days if they are stored in an airtight container in the refrigerator

Reheat:
Reheating leftovers in the microwave or on the stove top

 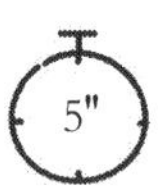 

5 | 5" | 11"

10.9 Ground Beef Skillet

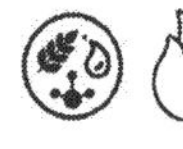 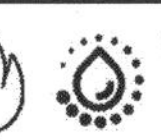 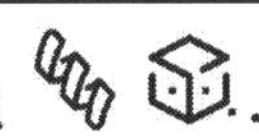 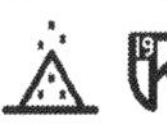 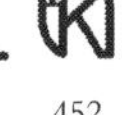

per serving	251 Cal	11.5g	11.3g	26.1g	4.2g		452 mg

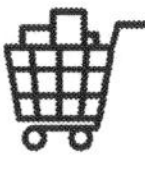

- Pureed pumpkin -2 cups
- Ground beef, preferably grass-fed -1 pound
- Ground black pepper -1/8 teaspoon
- Baby kale -5 ounces
- Salt -1/2 teaspoon

1. A big skillet should be heated at medium-high.
2. Use a wooden spoon to break up the ground beef before adding it to the skillet. For around 6 minutes, rotate the meat chunks every 2 minutes.
3. Include pumpkin. To blend, stir. Beef must be cooked for an additional 2 to 3 minutes.
4. Stir in the kale and seasonings. Cook kale for 1 minute, or until it barely wilts.

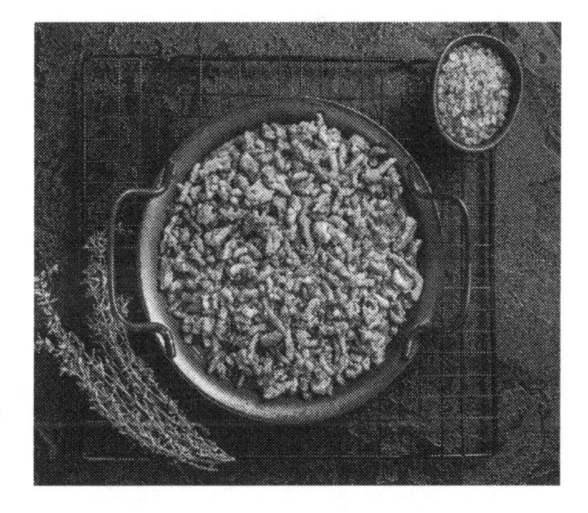

Storage:
Up to 3 days if they are stored in an airtight container in the refrigerator. (By the way, this is a fantastic lunch to bring to work.)

Reheat:
Reheating leftovers in the microwave or on the stove top

10.10 Chili con carne

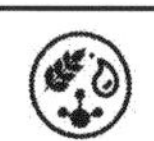 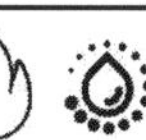 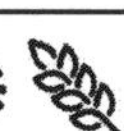 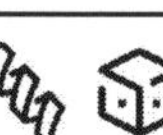 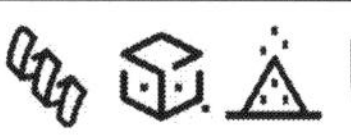 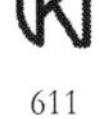

per serving	324 Cal	8.3g	20g	40.1g	1.9g	611 mg

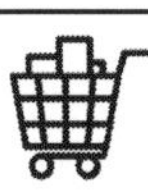

- Garlic-infused oil -2 tbsp
- Beef mince - 500 g
- Oregano -1 teaspoon
- Crushed Chile paste, 1 teaspoon (or chili powder)
- Salt and black pepper taste
- Bell pepper, -1
- Spring onion stalks (only the green part) -2
- Cumin -3/4 teaspoon
- Tomato puree -1-tablespoon
- Canned tomato cubes- 400 gram
- Beef broth (chicken or vegetables are also acceptable); just make sure it's low FODMAP -150 ml
- Green beans -1/2 cup
- Ground paprika -1/2 teaspoon

1. A big pot should be heated at medium heat. When heated, add the oil and the beef mince and cook over medium heat. Add the crushed chili paste or chili powder, cumin, oregano, and ground paprika. Add salt and pepper, then continue cooking until the meat turns brown.
2. Cut the spring onion into rings and the bell pepper into chunks. They should be added to the ground meat and cooked for an additional few minutes.
3. On low heat, add the tomato puree, diced tomatoes, and broth; simmer for about 10 minutes.
4. The beans should be rinsed, drained, and added to the pan. Cook on low heat for 10 more minutes.
5. Taste, if you like it spicier, add more chili powder or paste.
6. Serve with rice, quinoa, or pasta.

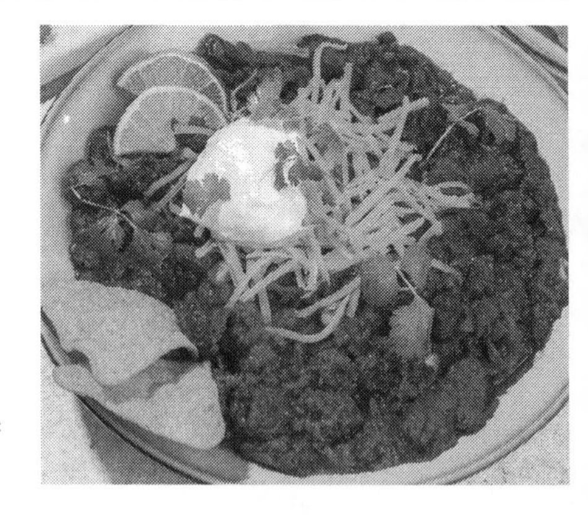

Storage:
Up to 3 days if they are stored in an airtight container in the refrigerator. (By the way, this is a fantastic lunch to bring to work.)

Reheat:
Reheating leftovers in the microwave or on the stove top

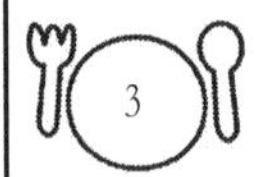 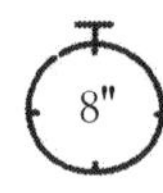 

10.11 Ground Beef Picadillo

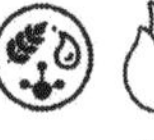  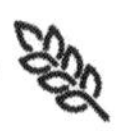 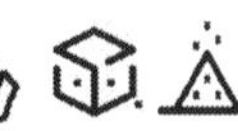 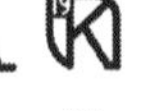

per serving	333 Cal	9.4g	26.3g	36g	7.6g	511 mg

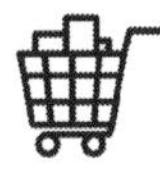

- 1 pound of lean ground beef.
- Red wine vinegar, 2 teaspoons
- can of crushed tomatoes – 3.5 cups
- Chopped red bell pepper -1.
- pitted green olives in a half-cup
- Capers, 1/4 cup
- Raisins -3 tbsp.
- Cumin powder -1 tablespoon
- 1 bay leaf, 2

1. Cook the ground beef for 7-8 minutes, or until browned, in a large skillet over medium-high heat.
2. Cook the potatoes and bell pepper for an additional five minutes, or until the vegetables begin to soften (everything does not need to be fully cooked yet).
3. Tomatoes, red wine vinegar, cumin, oregano, and bay leaves should all be added. Then, cover the pan and let it simmer for 30 minutes on medium-low heat.
4. Add the raisins, olives, capers, salt, and black pepper, and simmer uncovered for a further 15 minutes.

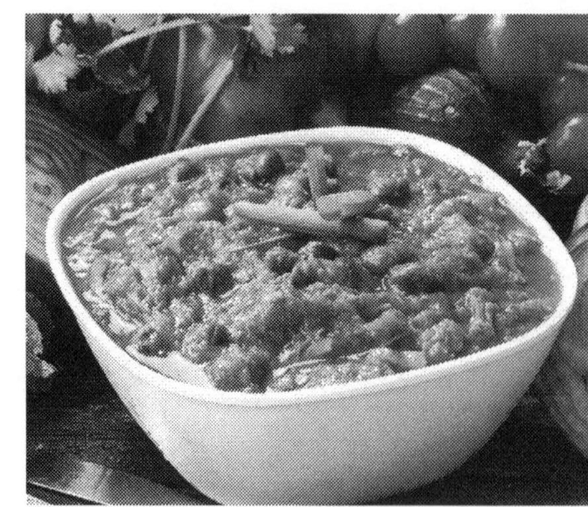

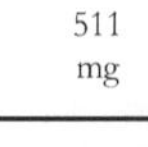

Storage:
Up to 3 days if they are stored in an airtight container in the refrigerator. (By the way, this is a fantastic lunch to bring to work.)

Reheat:
Reheating leftovers in the microwave or on the stove top

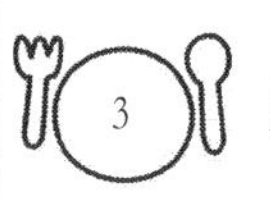

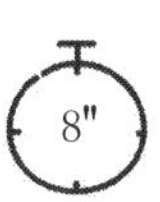

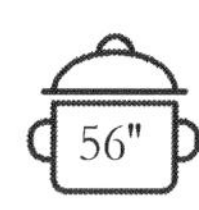

10.12 Goulash

 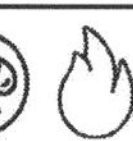 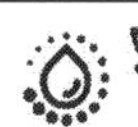 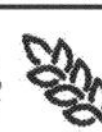 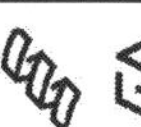 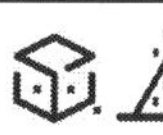 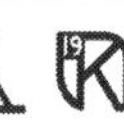

per serving | 538 Cal | 14.2g | 44.3g | 57.5g | 11g | 511 mg

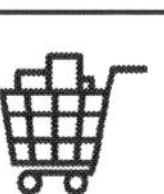

- Ground turkey or beef -2 pounds
- Shredded Cheddar Cheese, 1/2 cup
- Water -1/2 cup
- Garlic infused oil -1/3 cup
- 2 (15-ounce) tomato sauce cans
- Chopped tomatoes -15-ounce cans
- Low FODMAP Tuscan Herb Seasoning, 1 tablespoon
- Low-FODMAP adobo seasoning -1 tablespoon
- Bay leaves -3
- To taste, salt
- Black pepper, 1/2 tsp.
- Uncooked elbow macaroni without gluten -2 cups
- Shredded Mozzarella Cheese, 1/2 cup
- Low FODMAP beef broth - 1/2 cup

1. Cook your ground meat in a big skillet over medium-high heat until half done, then turn off the heat.
2. To fully cook the meat, add the oil, turn the heat back on, and stir.
3. Add the following ingredients: water, broth, tomato sauce, diced tomatoes, bay leaves, low FODMAP Tuscan Herb Seasoning, salt, and low FODMAP adobo Seasoning. Mix well.
4. Reduce heat, then cover. Cook for about 20 minutes, stirring every so often.
5. Stir well to incorporate after adding the uncooked gluten-free elbow macaroni to the skillet.
6. Recover the lid once again, and simmer for around 30 minutes.
7. After cooking, take off the bay leaves.
8. Cheddar cheese is the sole addition; combine.
9. Just before serving, add the mozzarella.

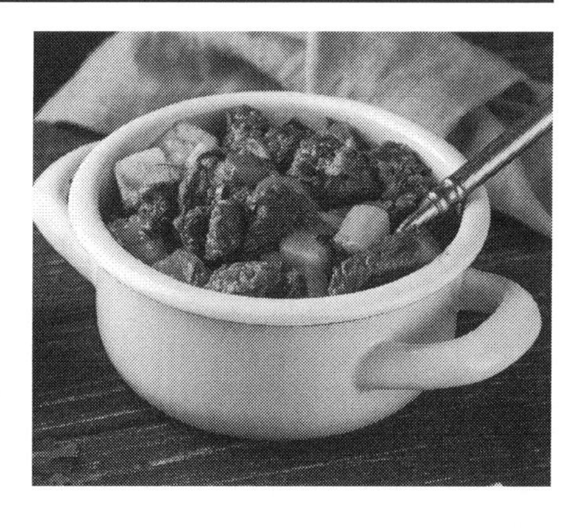

Storage:
Up to 3 days if they are stored in an airtight container in the refrigerator. (By the way, this is a fantastic lunch to bring to work.)

Reheat:
Reheating leftovers in the microwave or on the stove top

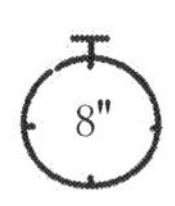

10.13 Pork Paella

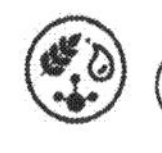 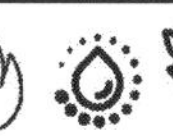 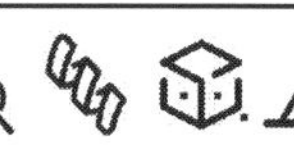 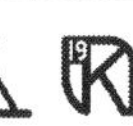

per serving | 538 Cal | 14.2g | 44.3g | 57.5g | 11g | 511 mg

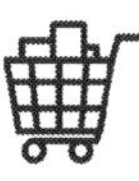

- Smoked paprika, 1 teaspoon
- Garlic infused oil of -2 teaspoons
- Boneless, thinly sliced, bite-sized slices of pork loin - 1 1/2 pounds
- Low FODMAP broth. -1 1/2 cups
- Diced tomatoes -1 cup
- Turmeric, ground 1 teaspoon
- Dry thyme 1/2 tsp.
- Green onion tops, cut into half a cup (green parts only)
- Red bell pepper, chopped, 1 cup
- Brown rice cooked, 2 cups

1. Garlic-infused olive oil in a large skillet should be heated to a medium-high temperature. For 8 minutes, or until almost done, cook the boneless pork loin strips. Red bell pepper is added, stirred, and cooked for two more minutes.
2. The skillet needs to be filled with brown rice, low FODMAP broth , diced tomatoes, paprika, turmeric, and thyme. Stir to combine. mixture is heated until it boils. Reduce heat to medium, cover, and simmer for 12 minutes while stirring occasionally. When the liquid has almost completely been absorbed, remove the lid and simmer for a further five minutes.
3. Just the green tops of the green onions should be added to the paella mixture. Warm up and add any desired garnishes.

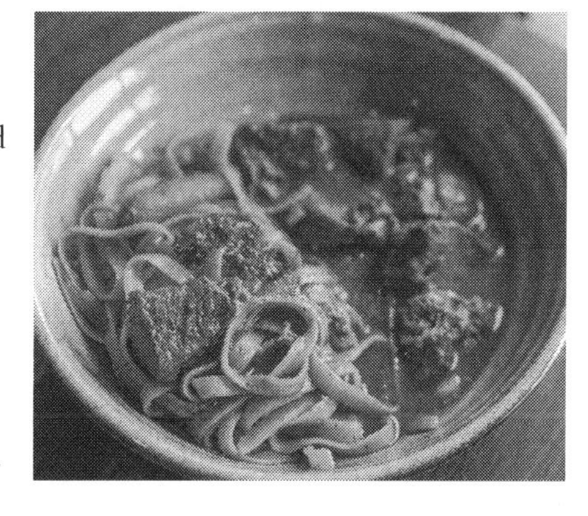

Storage:
Up to 3 days if they are stored in an airtight container in the refrigerator. (By the way, this is a fantastic lunch to bring to work.)

Reheat:
Reheating leftovers in the microwave or on the stove top

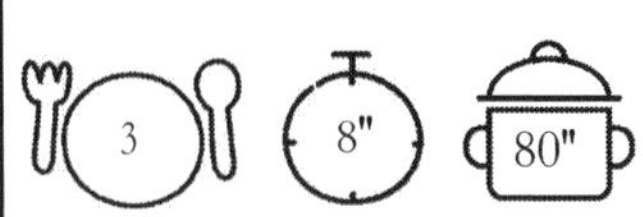

10.14 Baked Pork Chops

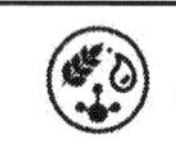 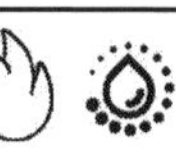 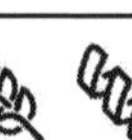 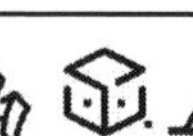 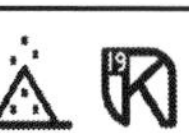

per serving 538 Cal 14.2g 44.3g 57.5g 11g 511 mg

- Boneless pork chops of - 4
- ½ cup of low-FODMAP chicken stock or broth (or water)
- Salt and pepper each of 1/4 tsp.
- Dried chives 2 tsp.
- Garlic-Infused Oil, 1 tablespoon
- 1 tablespoon of dried parsley
- Dried sage 1/2 tsp.
- Unsalted butter - 1 tablespoon

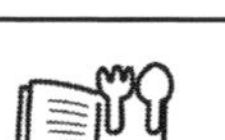

1. Oven temperature of 350 °F. A 13" x 9" baking pan should be sprayed with cooking spray.
2. Pork chops are seasoned with salt and pepper on both sides before going into the pan. Equally distribute the chives, parsley, and sage. Sprinkle some garlic infused oil on top. Butter should be placed on top of each pork chop. Water, chicken stock, or broth should be added to the pan's bottom.
3. With the pan completely covered with foil, bake for one hour. Bake the pan uncovered for a further 15 to 20 minutes. Serve.

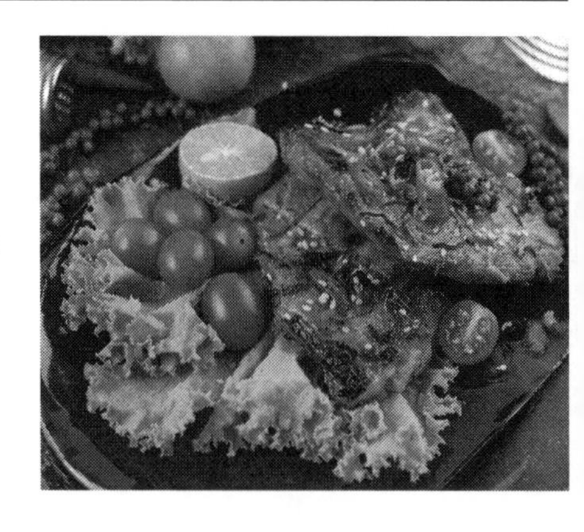

Storage:
Up to 3 days if they are stored in an airtight container in the refrigerator. (By the way, this is a fantastic lunch to bring to work.)

Reheat:
Reheating leftovers in the microwave or on the stove top

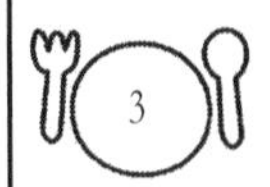 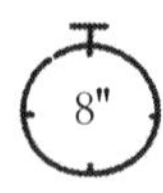 

10.15 Grilled Pork Chops with Lemon & Sage

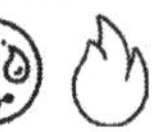 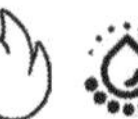 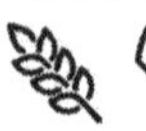 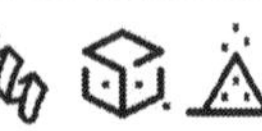 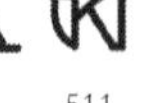

per serving 538 Cal 14.2g 44.3g 57.5g 11g 511 mg

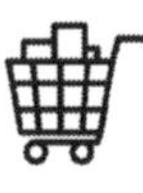

- Pork chops, bone-in or boneless 4

a low FODMAP Marinade for pork chops

- Salt, 1 1/2 teaspoons
- Lemon zest, 2 teaspoons,
- Dried chives 2 tbsp,
- Coarsely chopped fresh sage 1 tablespoon
- Garlic-Infused Oil, of 3 tbsp,
- Lemon juice, two tbsp,
- Black pepper, ground1 teaspoon
- Cayenne powder, crushed1 /4 teaspoon
- Extra virgin olive oil, 1 tablespoon

1. Before grilling, place the pork chops in a gallon-sized zip-top bag and let aside for at least two hours.
2. Add the ingredients for the pork chop marinade to a measuring cup or small bowl and whisk to combine. Place the pork chops, marinade, and plastic bag in a zip-top bag. To evenly sprinkle the coating over the pork chops, jiggle the bag with your hands. Marinate the bag for at least two hours in the refrigerator.
3. 400°F (204°C) on medium heat should be used to preheat the grill or grill pan (I use and adore a natural gas grill). Put the pork chops on the grill and discard any marinade that is left over.

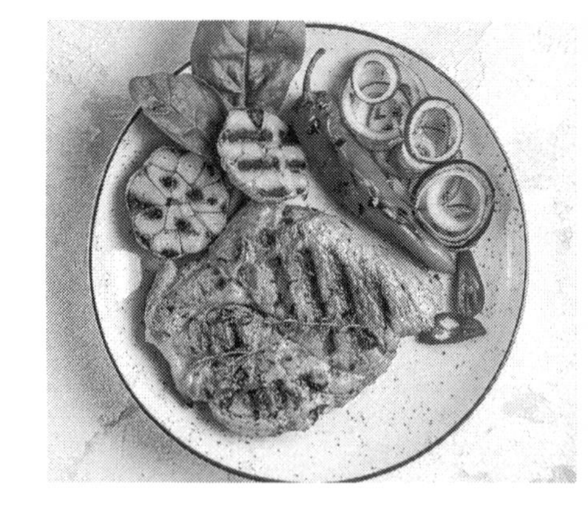

Storage:
Up to 3 days if they are stored in an airtight container in the refrigerator. (By the way, this is a fantastic lunch to bring to work.)

Reheat:
Reheating leftovers in the microwave or on the stove top

CHAPTER 11

SNACKS RECIPES

 14 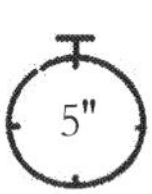 5"  18"

11.1 Chocolate-dipped dried figs

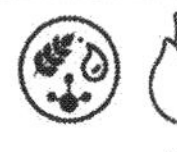 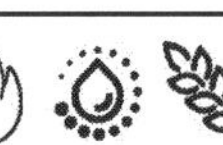 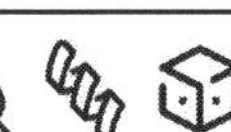 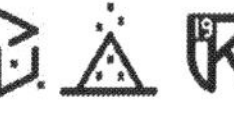 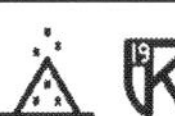

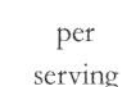 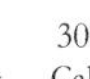 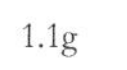 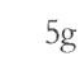

per serving	30 Cal	1.1g	5g	0.4g	1g		2 mg

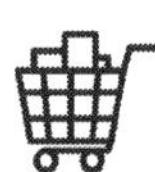

- Chips of dark chocolate -1/4 cup
- Macadamia nuts, finely chopped -1 tbsp.
- Dried California figs -8
- Coconut oil -1/2 tsp.

1. Put parchment paper on a little baking sheet. The California Dried Figs' stems should be cut off and discarded. The dried figs should be cut in half lengthwise.
2. In a small microwave-safe bowl, combine the coconut oil and dark chocolate chips. until the chocolate is melted and smooth, microwave in increments of 20 seconds, stirring after each increment.
3. Grab the top of a fig that has been cut in half (where the stem was removed) and dip the dried fig approximately 12 to 23 into the molten chocolate. Place the chocolate-covered fig half on the baking sheet that has been prepared with parchment after gently shaking off any excess chocolate. Continue by using the remaining fig halves.
4. On the melted chocolate portion of the dipped fig, scatter chopped macadamia nuts.
5. The chocolate will firm if you freeze the chocolate-covered figs for around five minutes. Take away and serve.

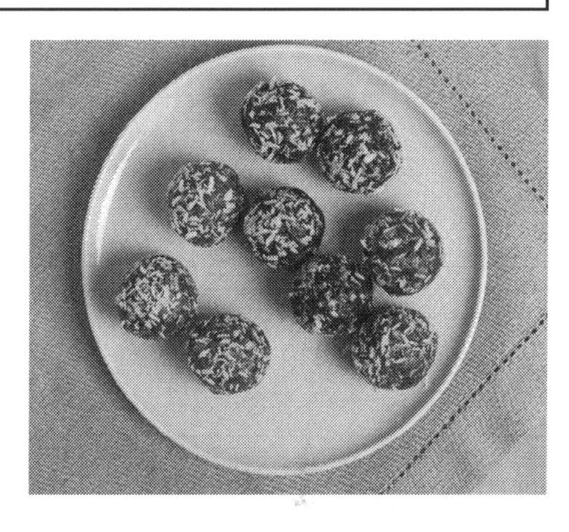

Storage:
The chocolate will firm if you freeze the chocolate-covered figs for around five minutes. Take away and serve.

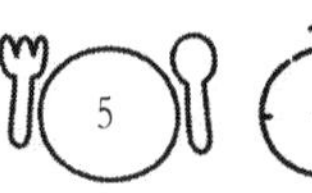 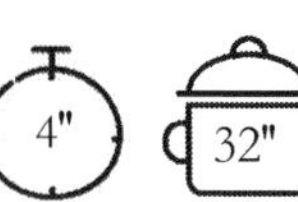 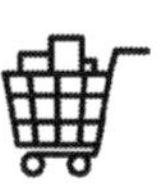

5 | 4" | 32"

11.2 French Fries

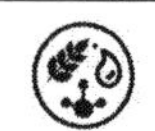 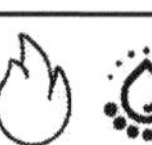 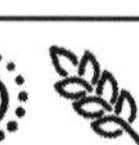 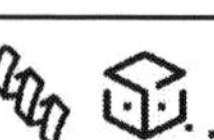 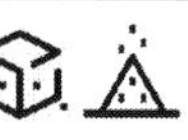 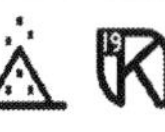

per serving	145 Cal	3g	27.5g	4g	2.1g	702 mg

- Washing and slicing into 1/2" fried strips 4 medium russet potatoes
- Olive oil, 1 tbsp

SEASONING MIX

- Dried rosemary- 0.5 teaspoon
- Salt ½ tsp
- Dried thyme -0.5 teaspoon
- Pepper -1/4 tsp

1. Set the oven's temperature to 400.
2. Washing and slicing potatoes
3. In a large bowl, place the sliced potatoes, drizzle with olive oil, Combine the seasoning ingredients in a separate bowl, then pour half of the seasoning mixture to the bowl of potatoes. Toss the potatoes one more to coat. The remaining seasoning mixture should be set aside.
4. The potato slices should be placed cut side down on a parchment-lined baking sheet, uniformly spaced apart, and without any overlap.

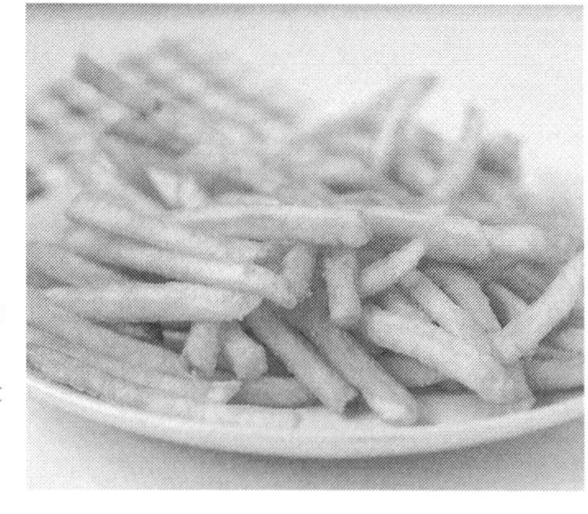

Storage:
Store into air tight container

Reheat:
Use microwave for reheat

11 | 14" | 48"

11.3 Banana Bread

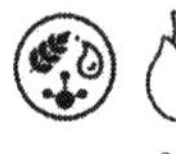  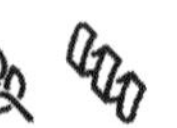 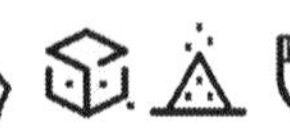 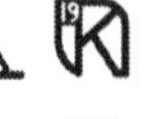

per serving	213 Cal	8g	35.2g	3.2g	18g	227 mg

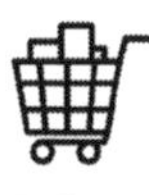

- Baking Soda - 1 teaspoon,
- Brown sugar - 100 g (1/2 cup)
- Dairy-free spread (butter or olive oil spread) -120 g (1/2 cup)
- 2 large eggs (lightly beaten)
- Vanilla extract -0.5 teaspoons
- Unripe bananas, -4
- Baking powder -1 teaspoon
- Salt -1/2 teaspoon
- Mixed spices -1/2 teaspoon
- Gluten-free all-purpose flour, - 210 g (1 1/2 cups)
- Lemon juice -2 tbsp,
- White sugar -52 g (1/4 cup)

1. Set the bake function on the oven to 180°C (355°F). Make a loaf pan lined or greased.
2. Bananas should be chopped into small pieces and microwaved for 30 seconds (this will help soften the firm bananas and make them easier to mash). Bananas should then be mashed till smooth.
3. Both Sugar and dairy free spread (or butter) are combined in a cream. Eggs, mashed banana, and vanilla extract should all be combined.
4. Mix the flour, salt, mixed spices, and baking powder in a bowl. Lemon juice and baking soda should be combined in a small cup (doing so will mask the baking soda's flavor and prevent your banana bread from tasting soapy).
5. Combine the wet components before adding the flour mixture and baking soda combination.
6. Place in the loaf pan and bake in the center of the oven for 45 minutes. If necessary, cook the loaf for a further five minutes after checking to see if the top is brown and the center comes out mostly clean.
7. If you want to enjoy your slice of banana bread warm, reheat it in the microwave for 20 to 30 seconds.

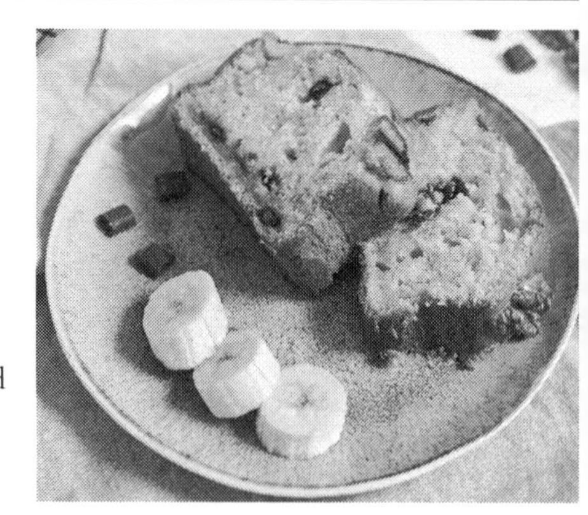

Storage:
Store into air tight container

Reheat:
use microwave for reheat

 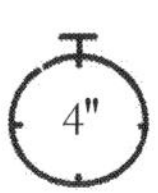 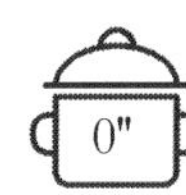

5 | 4" | 0"

11.4 Chocolate chia pudding mousse

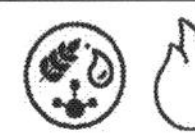 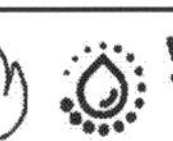 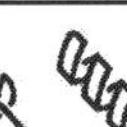 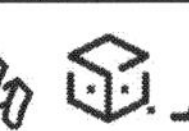 
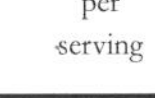 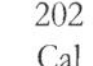

per serving	202 Cal	11.8g	20.7g	4.6g	9.8g	287 mg

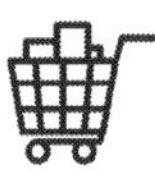

- Maple syrup -1/4 cup
- Coconut milk – 2 cups
- ½ cup chia seeds
- ¼ cup of cocoa powder or cacao powder
- Vanilla extract -1 teaspoon

1. Into a powerful blender, add all the components.
2. The pudding should be creamy after one minute of high-speed blending.
3. In a bowl, transfer the pudding, cover, and chill for at least four hours.
4. With a dollop of coconut whipped cream, chocolate shavings, and chopped almonds, serve the chocolate chia mousse.

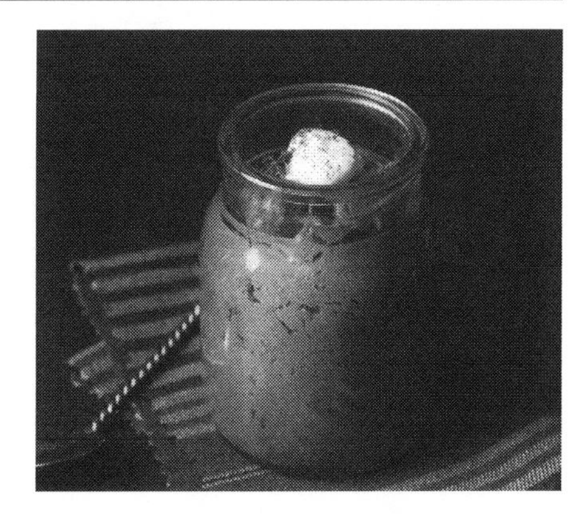

Storage:
Store into air tight container

 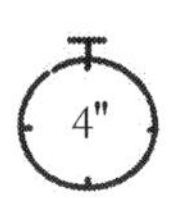 

5 | 4" | 8"

11.5 Salted Margarita Popcorn

 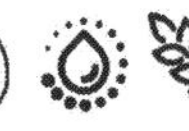 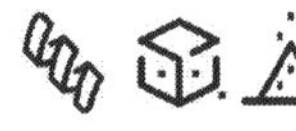 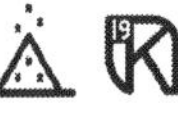 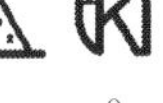

per serving	132 Cal	7.8g	15.3g	2.7g	0g	0 mg

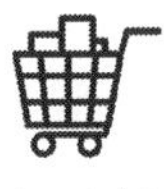

- Sea salt -1/4 teaspoon
- Melted coconut oil -2 tbsp
- Lime zest -1
- Popcorn kernels, 1/3 cup

1. On a medium-high heat, melt 1 1/2 tbsp of the coconut oil in a saucepan.
2. Add 1 kernel of popcorn and reduce the heat to medium. When the kernel bursts, the oil is hot enough to add the remaining ingredients.
3. While occasionally shaking the pot, add the remaining kernels. Once all of the kernels have popped, turn off the heat and stir in the remaining 1/2 tbsp coconut oil, sea salt, and lime zest. (This will prevent the bottom kernels from burning.)
4. Serve right away.

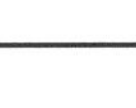

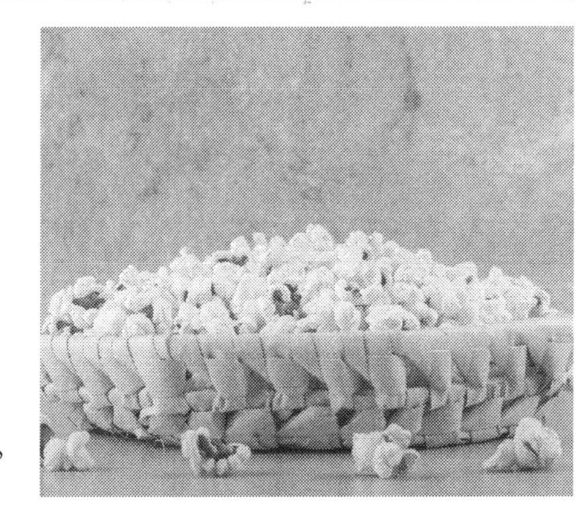

Storage:
Store into air tight container

11.6 Baked Egg Cups

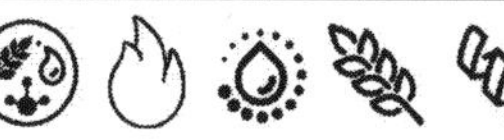

per serving	74 Cal	5.1g	0.4g	6.3g	0.3g	58 mg

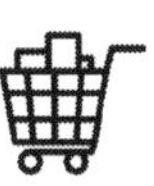

- Almond milk unsweetened -1/4 cup
- Salt -1/2 tsp.
- Finely chopped fresh spinach- 3/4 cup
- Diced around a quarter of a large red bell pepper
- Eggs -5
- Ground black pepper -1/4 tsp.

1. Set the oven to 350°F.
2. Apply olive oil to the muffin tin and set it aside.
3. In medium bowl whisk together eggs, unsweetened almond milk, salt and pepper.
4. Take muffin tin and add a spoonful. To each muffin tin, add a tablespoon of sliced bell pepper and a tablespoon of ripped spinach.
5. Filling in the space at the top, pour the egg mixture over the top (it will expand and rise as it is cooking – but then will deflate once it cools).
6. 17 minutes will be needed to cook in the oven.
7. If the very top isn't entirely done when you take it out of the oven, put it back in for additional 2-3 minutes.

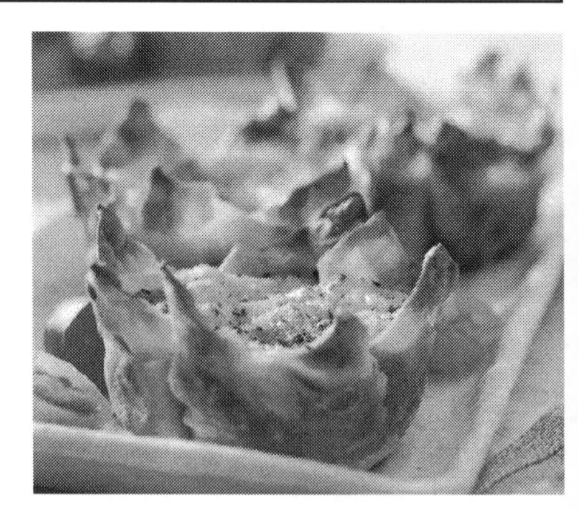

Storage:
For up to four days, keep in the refrigerator in an airtight container.

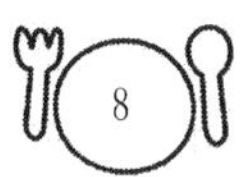 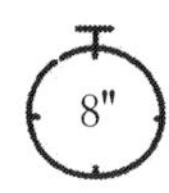 

11.7 Chocolate Chip Cookies

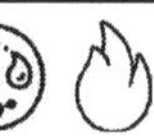 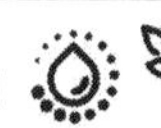 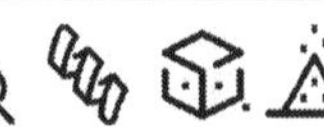 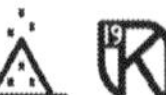

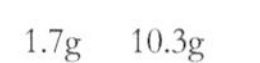

per serving	123 Cal	5.7g	18.4g	1.7g	10.3g	1 mg

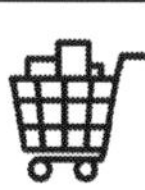

- Coconut sugar – ½ cup
- Vanilla extract -1 tsp.
- Water – 2 tbsp.
- Sea salt, fine -0.5 teaspoons
- ½ teaspoon of baking soda
- Buckwheat flour -1 cup
- 1 teaspoon of apple cider vinegar
- Dark chocolate chips, half a cup
- Melted coconut oil, 1/3 cup

1. Set the oven to 350 degrees Fahrenheit and line a large baking sheet with silicone mat or parchment paper.
2. Mix the buckwheat flour, coconut sugar, water, oil, vanilla extract, salt, and baking soda in a large bowl. The vinegar will then be added, reacting with the baking soda to give the cookies a slight rise.
3. When the dough is uniformly divided into 12 mounds on the prepared baking sheet, fold in the chocolate chips. Since these cookies won't spread much, flatten each one with your palms. At 350°F, bake for about 10 minutes or until the edges are crisp. At least 10 minutes should pass before serving.

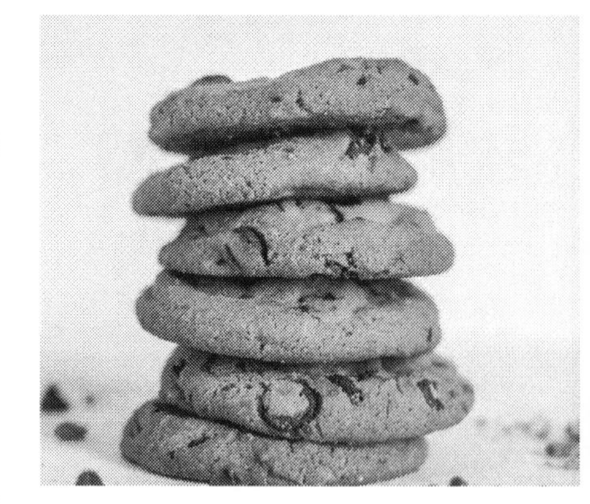

Storage:
For up to four days, keep in the refrigerator in an airtight container.

 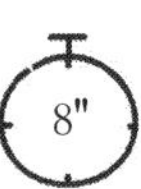 

21 | 8" | 0"

11.8 Peanut Butter Brownie Bites

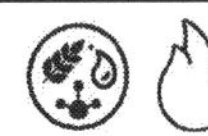 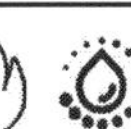 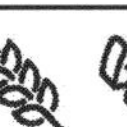 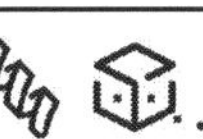 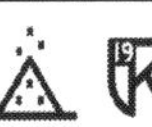 

per serving	123 Cal	5.7g	18.4g	1.7g	10.3g		1 mg

- Chia seeds, 2 tbsp.
- Unsweetened peanut butter, which is 1/2 cup.
- Pure maple syrup -1/4 cup
- Cocoa powder, 2 tsp.
- Rolled oats, 1 cup (use gluten-free rolled oats for gluten-free)
- Salt -1/4 tsp.
- Mini Chocolate Chips, 1/4 cup

1. Put peanut butter and oats in a food processor. Once the oats and peanut butter are barely combined and coarsely ground, pulse. Several repetitions ought to accomplish the trick.
2. Add the cocoa powder, chia seeds, 1/4 cup maple syrup, chocolate chips, and (optional) salt. Pulse to thoroughly combine. If the mixture looks too dry, add a tablespoon at a time additional maple syrup to reach the ideal, somewhat sticky, rollable consistency. The consistency will vary according on the type of peanut butter used.
3. Grab a small bit of the mixture between your clean hands, squeeze it together, and roll it into a ball that is about the size of an inch. Repeat with the remainder of the mixture, placing the ball on a pan coated with paper.
4. Place the completed item in the freezer until it becomes non-stick. Place in a freezer-safe container for storing after transfer. Although they can be kept in the refrigerator to eat, wait a moment or two for the food to thaw (if frozen).

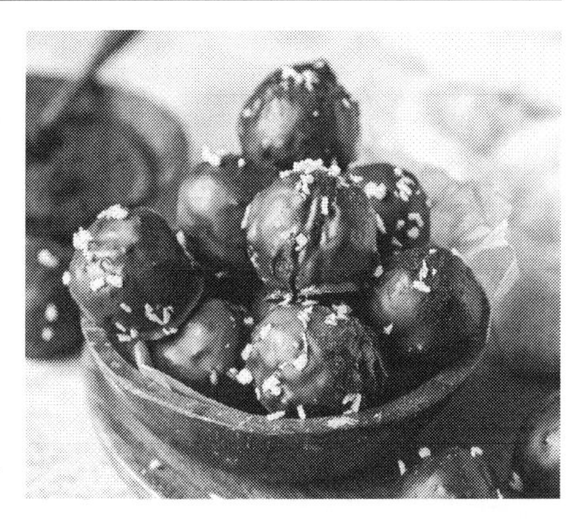

Storage:
Place in a freezer-safe container for storing after transfer. Although they can be kept in the refrigerator

3 | 110" | 0"

11.9 Matcha Chia Pudding

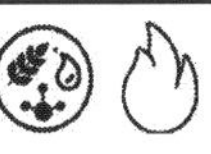 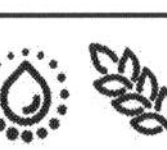 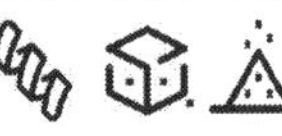 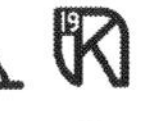 

per serving	184 Cal	8.7g	28.4g	1.3g	20.3g		82 mg

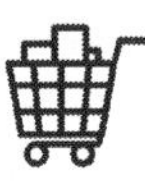

- Matcha green tea powder, 1 heaping teaspoon
- Coconut yoghurt, 2 tbsp,
- Chia seeds, whole – ¼ cup
- Pure vanilla extract, 1 teaspoon
- Maple syrup, pure-2 teaspoons
- Coconut milk -1 1/4 cups

1. Divide the chia seeds into three small jars or Tupperware containers
2. Between the jars/containers, distribute the coconut milk, coconut yogurt, vanilla extract, maple syrup, and matcha.
3. Shake the jars or containers for 10 to 20 seconds after carefully fastening the lids.
4. Place in the refrigerator for an hour to set.
5. Give the matcha chia pudding another thorough shake and refrigerate for at least another hour after the first hour.
6. Enjoy as is or top with a dollop of coconut yoghurt and fresh berries once cooled and thickened into a pudding consistency!

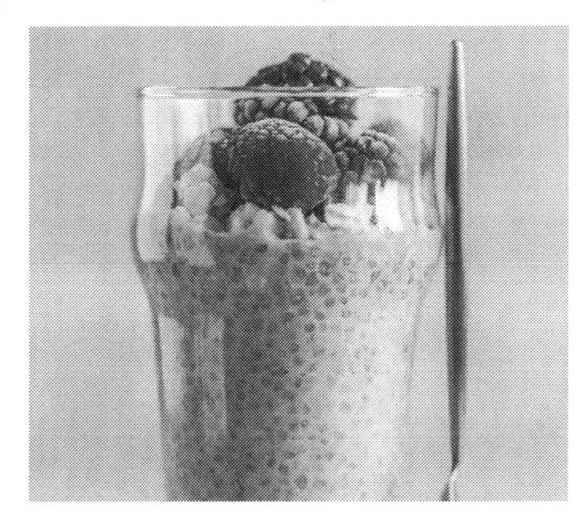

Storage:
Place in a freezer-safe container for storing after transfer. Although they can be kept in the refrigerator

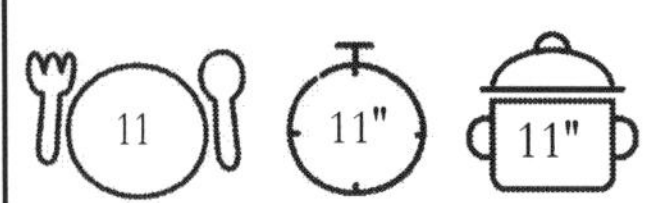
11 11" 11"

11.10 Deviled Eggs

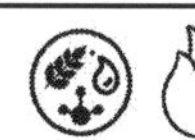 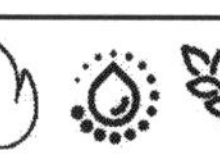 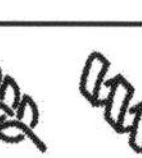 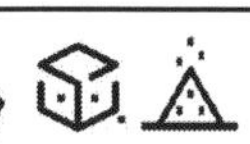 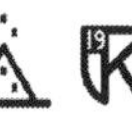

per serving	78 Cal	5.7g	1.9g	4.3g	0.9g		59 mg

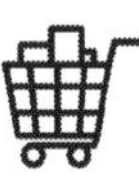

- Cooled and peeled hard-boiled eggs -6
- Mayo – 3 tbsp.
- Salt, and pepper, to taste
- Cooked and crumbled bacon slices -2
- Diced chives – 1 tbsp.
- Dijon mustard, 1 tsp.

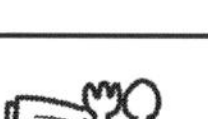

1. Preparation
2. The hard boiled eggs should be cut in half lengthwise. Set the egg whites on a dish and use a spoon to scoop out the yolk and place it in a small bowl.
3. With a fork, mash the yolks and stir in the salt, pepper, Dijon mustard, mayo. Everything must be combined and stirred until creamy.
4. Put some of the Deviled egg mixture back into each egg white's hole using a spoon.
5. Add a substantial amount of bacon bits and a few chives as garnish.

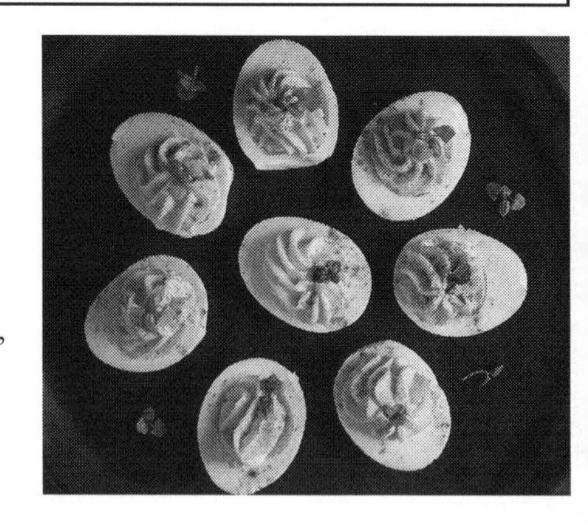

Storage:
Place in a freezer-safe container for storing after transfer. Although they can be kept in the refrigerator

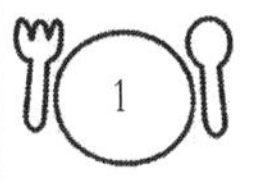  
1 11" 0"

11.11 Raspberry Chia Jam

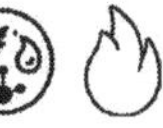 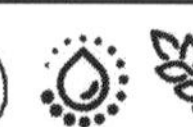 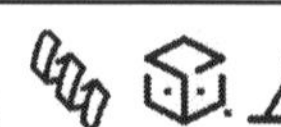 

per serving	98 Cal	3.3g	14.9g	3.5g	5.9g		134 mg

- Chia seeds, 1 tsp
- Pure maple syrup (or add more to taste) – 1 tsp.
- Raspberries – 10

1. Raspberries should be mashed with a fork in a small bowl until they resemble jam.
2. chia seeds and maple syrup have been added (adjusting to taste preferences).
3. Before serving, wait 10 minutes to give the chia seeds a chance to soften.

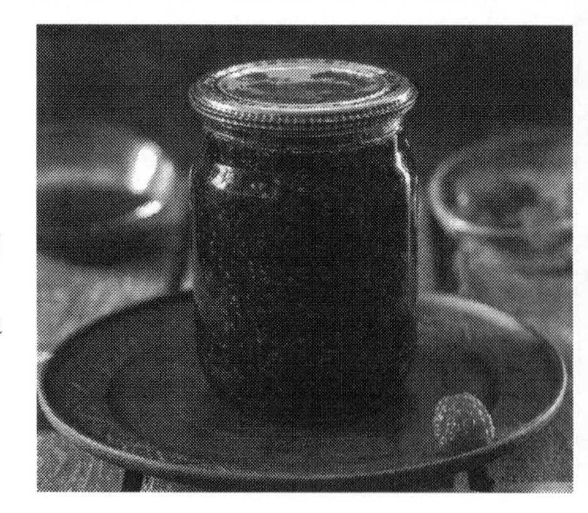

Storage:
Place in a freezer-safe container for storing after transfer. Although they can be kept in the refrigerator

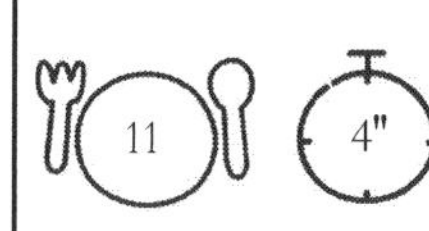

11.12 Pumpkin Seeds

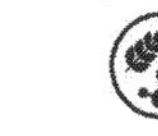 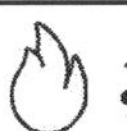 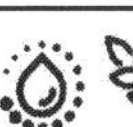 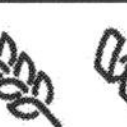 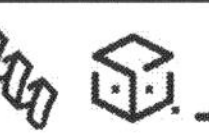 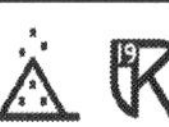 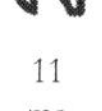

per serving	49 Cal	3.9g	3.1g	1.2g	2g	11 mg

- Ground nutmeg, 1/8 tsp.
- Pumpkin seed -1/2 cup
- melted butter -2 tbsp,
- Ground ginger -1/4 teaspoon
- Ground cinnamon, 1 teaspoon
- Ground cloves -1/8 teaspoon
- to taste, sea salt
- maple syrup - a teaspoon

1. Set the oven to 275°F. Use parchment paper to cover a baking sheet.
2. Pumpkin seeds should be put in a medium bowl. Add melted butter and maple syrup, then whisk to thoroughly cover the seeds.
3. Combine salt, Ground cinnamon, Ground ginger, Ground nutmeg, and Ground cloves in a small bowl. Stir the mixture into the seeds to coat them.
4. Cover the baking sheet with seeds. Stirring regularly, bake the seeds for 30 to 40 minutes, or until they are golden brown. Take out of the oven, then let cool before eating.

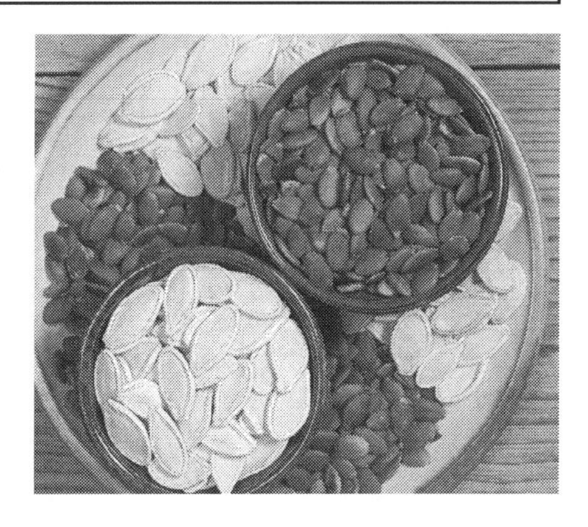

Storage:
Place in a freezer-safe container for storing after transfer. Although they can be kept in the refrigerator

11.13 Pomegranate Orange Salsa

 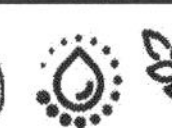 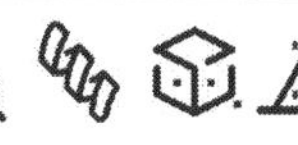 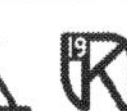

per serving	88 Cal	0.3g	22.6g	1.4g	19.1g	300 mg

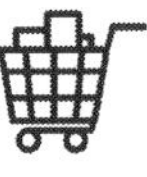

- Orange, sliced and segmented- 4
- Pomegranate seeds-1/2 cup
- Minced jalapeno (optional), - ½
- Finely minced cilantro leaves- ¼ cup
- Lime zest (optional)- ½ teaspoon
- ½ cup of lime juice
- Chopped green onions, only the green parts – 1/3 cup
- Maple syrup, 1 tablespoon
- Salt – ¼ teaspoon

1. Combine the diced orange, pomegranate seeds, green onion, minced jalapeno, cilantro leaves, lime zest, lime juice, maple syrup, salt, in a bowl. Mix well.
2. Serve as a dipping sauce for grilled fish, poultry, or shrimp or with corn chips.

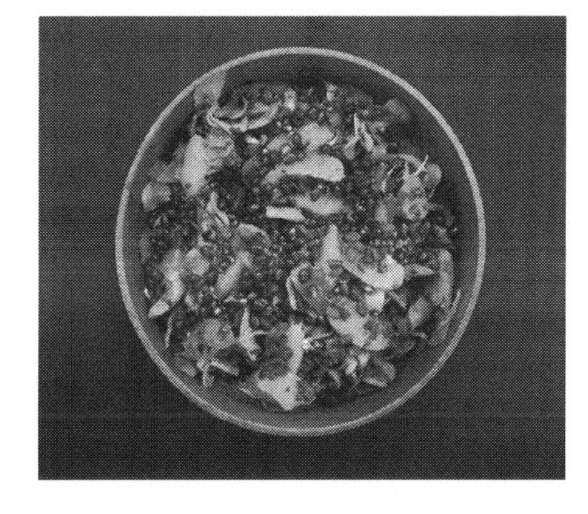

Storage:
Place in a freezer-safe container for storing after transfer. Although they can be kept in the refrigerator

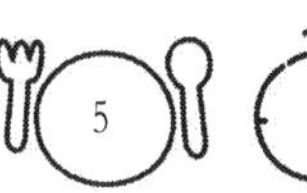

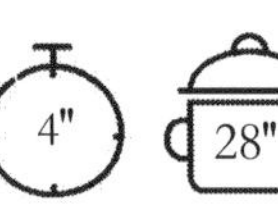

28"

11.14 Maple Walnut Granola

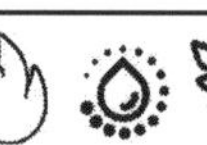
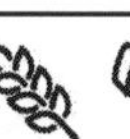
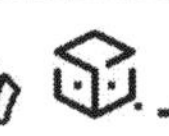

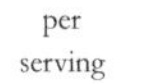
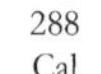

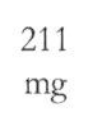

per serving	288 Cal	15g	13.2g	7.1g	10.8g		211 mg

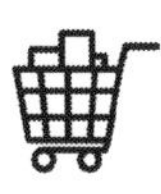

- Cinnamon powder- 1 tsp.
- Rolled oats, 2 cups
- Pure maple syrup- 1/3 cup
- Chunks of walnuts – ½ cup
- Chia seeds- 2 tsp.
- Melted coconut oil -4 ounces

1. Set the oven to 300 °F. Use parchment paper to cover a baking sheet.
2. Maple syrup, coconut oil that has been melted, and cinnamon are combined in a sizable bowl.
3. Oats, walnuts, and chia seeds are optional additions. Mix by stirring.
4. Spread mixture evenly across a baking sheet that has been lined.
5. Granola should be crunchy and golden brown after 30 minutes of baking, stirring halfway through. Take out of the oven, then let cool to room temperature.
6. Granola can be served chilled dairy free milk

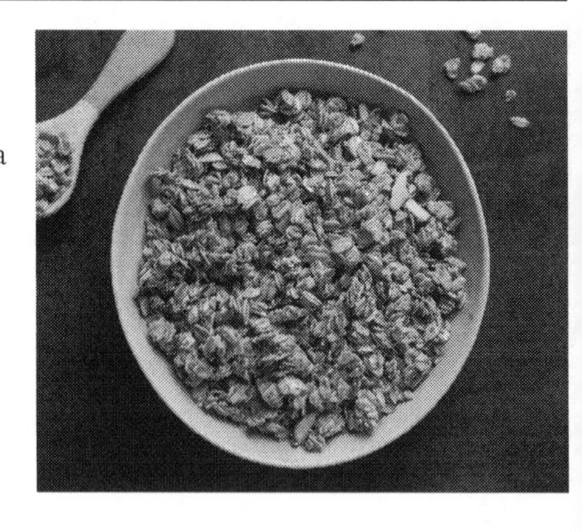

Storage:
Granola can be kept at room temperature for up to two weeks in an airtight container. For up to three months, freeze.

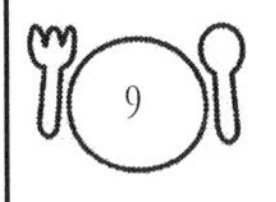

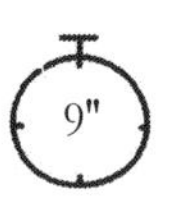

11.15 Red Pepper and Walnut Dip

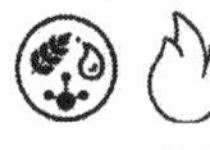

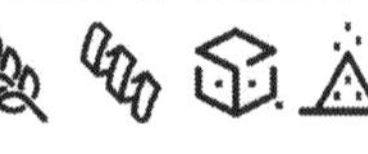
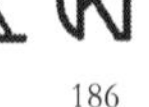

per serving	186 Cal	17.5g	4.7g	7g	1.8g		186 mg

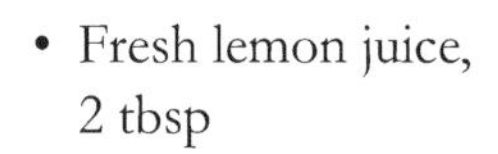

- Fresh lemon juice, 2 tbsp
- Red bell peppers in half lengthwise, removing the stems and seeds- 2
- Garlic-infused olive oil -2 tbsp.
- Cumin seeds -1/2 tsp.
- Pepper and salt
- Walnuts,- 1 1/2 cups

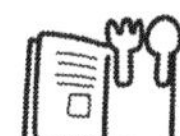

1. Set the oven to 450 degrees. A baking sheet with a rim should be lined with foil. The peppers should be roasted cut side down for 20 to 25 minutes, or until the skins are wrinkled and barely browned.
2. After removing from the oven, place in a bowl and allow to cool. After cooling for 30 minutes, wrap plastic wrap around the bowl.
3. Remove peppers from bowl after cooling. Put the bell pepper after removing the skins, walnuts, olive oil, lemon juice, and cumin into a food processor until smooth, process. Add salt and pepper to taste.
4. Serve dip with vegetables low in FODMAPs.

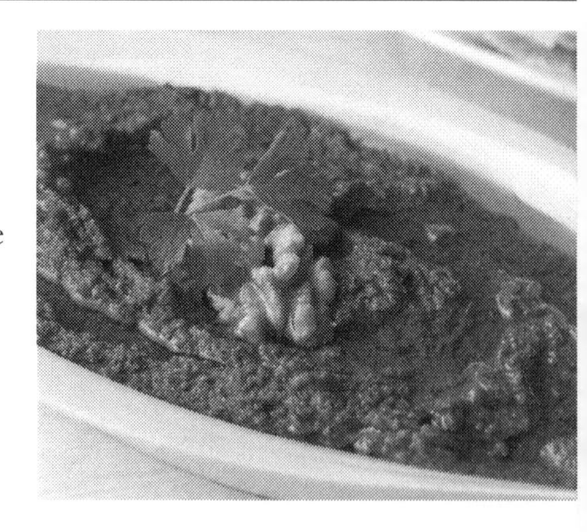

Storage:
For up to three days, store in the refrigerator in an airtight container.

CHAPTER 12

SMOOTHIES AND DRINKS RECIPES

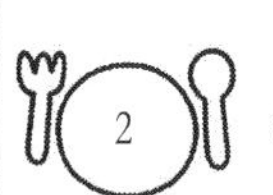 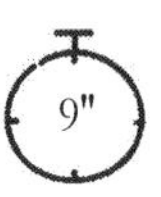 

12.1 Peanut & Banana Smoothie

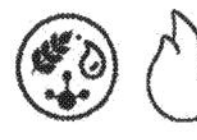 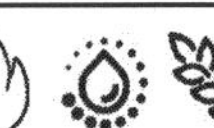 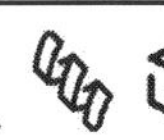 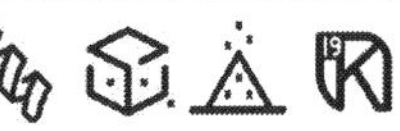 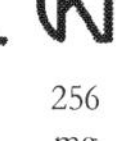

per serving	240 Cal	10.5g	34g	5.5g	24.8g		256 mg

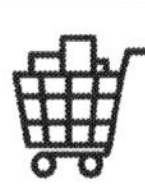

- Peanut butter -1 tablespoon
- Stevia - 1 tsp
- Unripe Banana - 1
- Coconut milk – 1cup
- Cinnamon - 1 teaspoon

1. In a blender or food processor, combine or process all ingredients until completely smooth

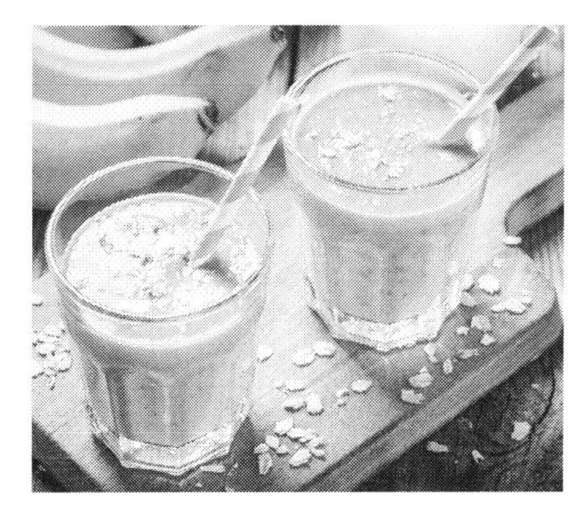

Storage:
For a maximum of three months, you can keep smoothies or their components in the freezer.

12.2 Blueberry Limeade

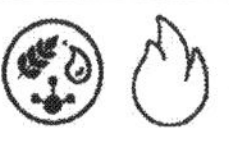 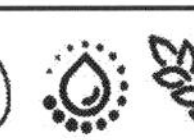 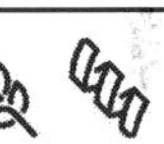 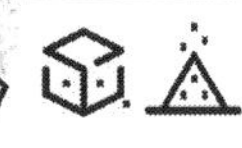 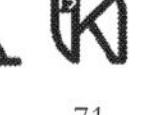

per serving	67 Cal	0.1g	18.4g	0.4g	13.4g		71 mg

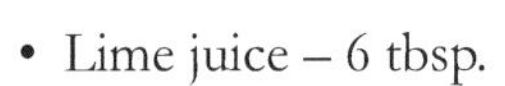

- Lime juice – 6 tbsp.
- Blueberries – 1 cup
- Ice cubes
- Sugar – 1/3 cup
- Water – 4 cups

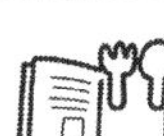

1. In a blender or food processor, combine or process all ingredients until completely smooth.

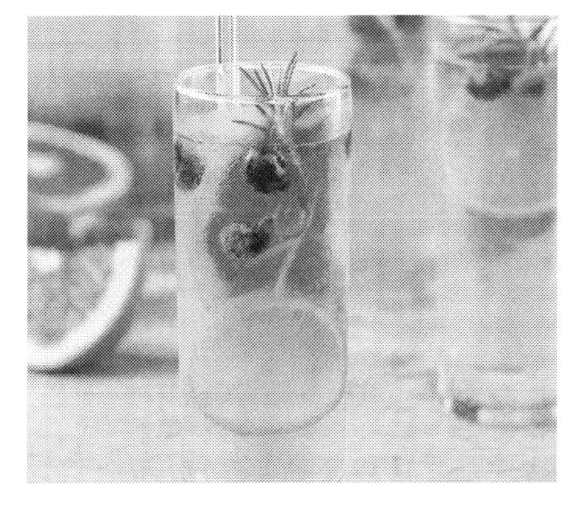

Storage:
For a maximum of three months, you can keep smoothies or their components in the freezer.

 2 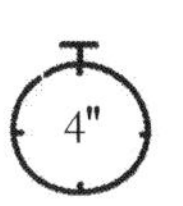 4"  0"

12.3 Blueberry & Chia Smoothie

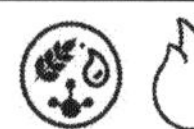 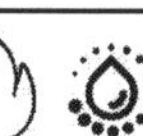 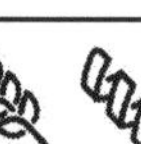 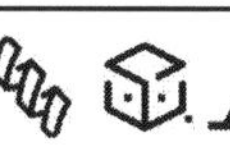 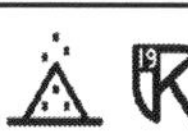

per serving	130 Cal	7g	17.6g	3g	7.3g	113 mg

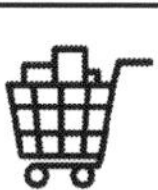

- Almond milk – 1-1/2 cups
- Ice cubes – 1 cup
- Blueberries – 1/3 cup
- Stevia – 1 tsp.
- Chia seeds – 1 tbsp

1. In a blender or food processor, combine or process all ingredients until completely smooth.

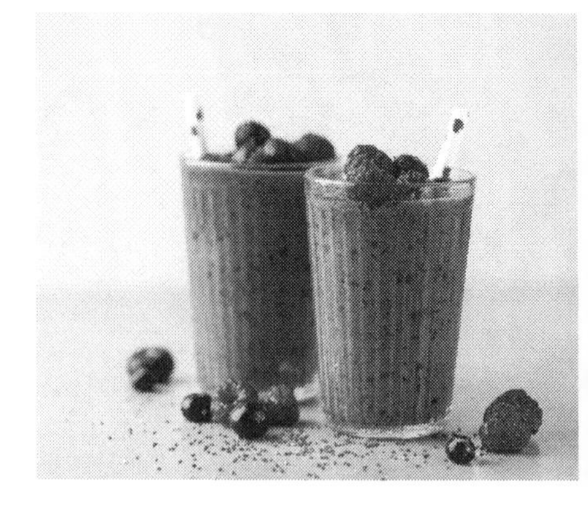

Storage:
For a maximum of three months, you can keep smoothies or their components in the freezer.

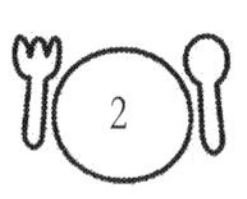 2 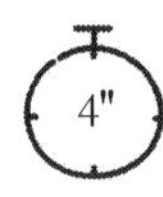 4" 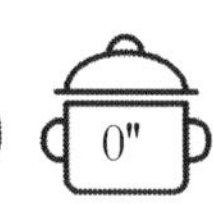 0"

12.4 Strawberry, Almond & Flax Smoothie

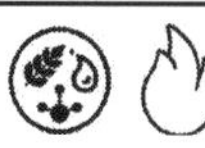  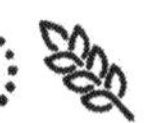 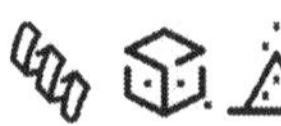 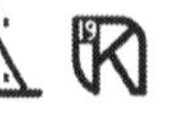

per serving	154 Cal	9.3g	16g	3.7g	7.8g	160 mg

- Almond butter -1 tbsp.
- fresh frozen strawberries – 1 cup
- Ice cubes – 1 cup
- flax seed meal– 1 tbsp.
- Stevia – 1 tsp.
- Almond milk – 1-1/2 cups

1. In a blender or food processor, combine or process all ingredients until completely smooth.

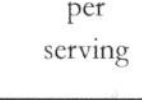

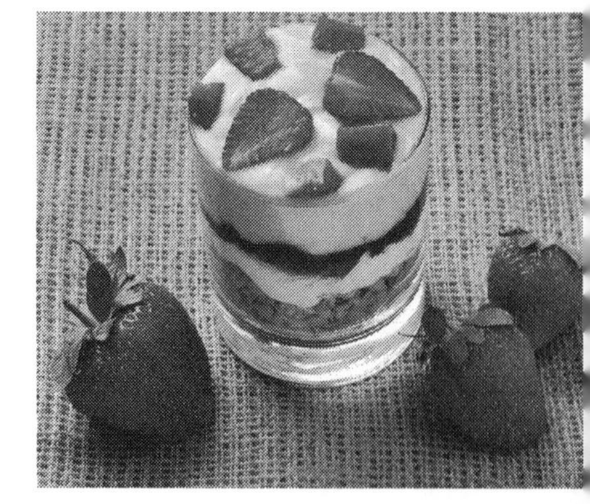

Storage:
For a maximum of three months, you can keep smoothies or their components in the freezer.

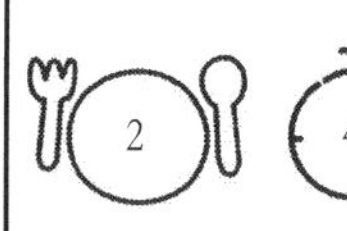 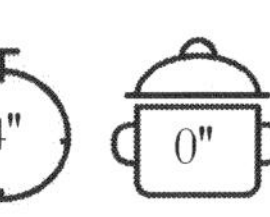 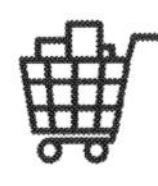

12.5 Green Smoothie

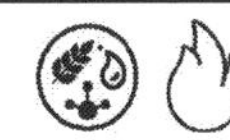 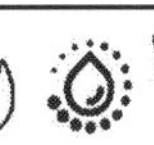 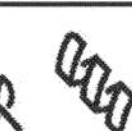 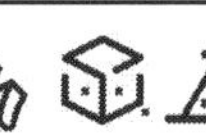 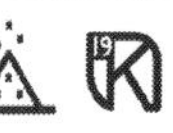

per serving	266 Cal	1.5g	53.6g	6.7g	7.8g		160 mg

- Unsweetened almond or coconut milk (or water) – 1 cup
- Kiwi -1
- Pineapple – 1cup
- Cucumber- 1
- Kale- 1 cup
- a pinch sea salt

1. In a blender or food processor, combine or process all ingredients until completely smooth.

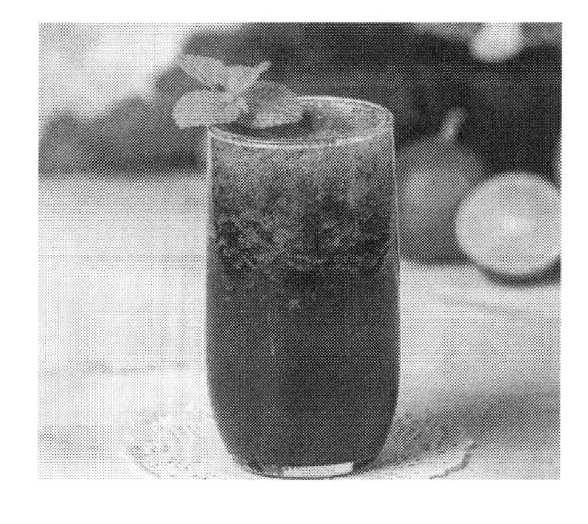

Storage:
For a maximum of three months, you can keep smoothies or their components in the freezer.

 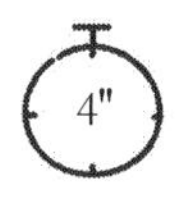 

12.6 Turmeric- Ginger Smoothie

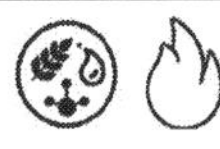 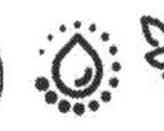 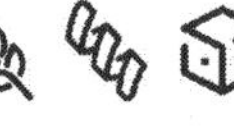 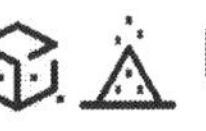 

per serving	167 Cal	7.5g	25.3g	3.1g	15g		455 mg

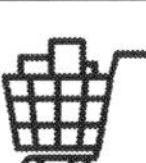

- Ground turmeric – ½ tsp.
- Kale – 1 cup
- Orange, peeled – 1
- Freshly ground pepper
- Water – 1 cup
- Unripe Banana – ½
- Coconut milk – ½ cup
- Fresh ginger – 1 tsp.

1. In a blender or food processor, combine or process all ingredients until completely smooth.

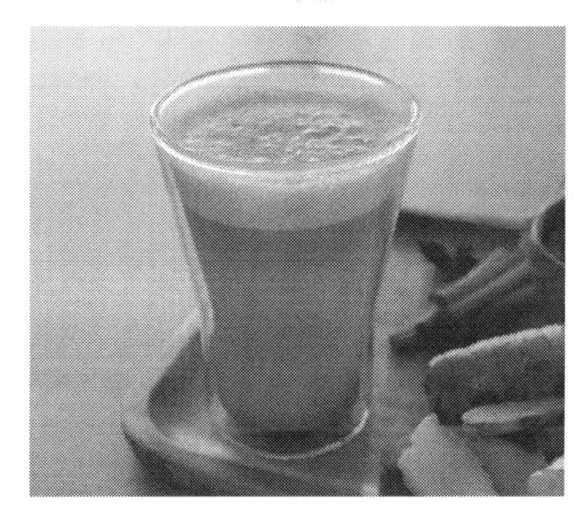

Storage:
For a maximum of three months, you can keep smoothies or their components in the freezer.

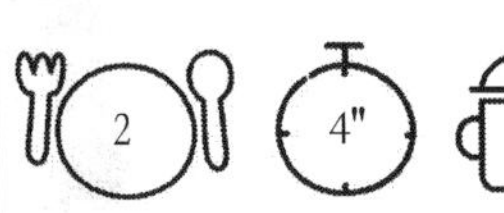

12.7 Kale Orange Smoothie

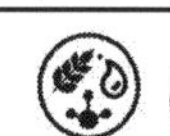 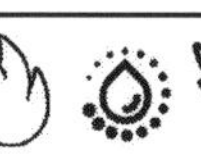 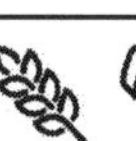 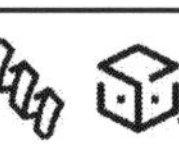 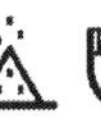

per serving	191 Cal	5.2g	34.7g	5g	20.6g	665 mg

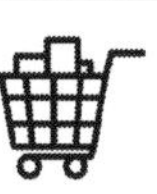

- Peanut butter – 1 tbsp.
- Orange, peeled – ½
- Coconut milk – 1 cup
- Unripe Banana, -1/2
- Kale leaves – 1 cup
- Maple syrup – 1 tbsp.

1. In a blender or food processor, combine or process all ingredients until completely smooth.

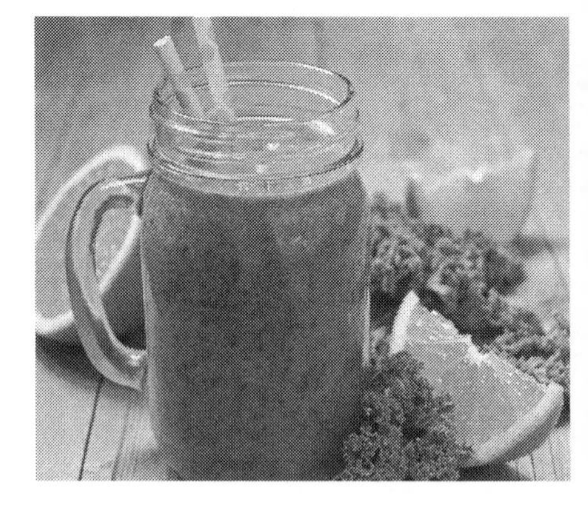

Storage:
For a maximum of three months, you can keep smoothies or their components in the freezer.

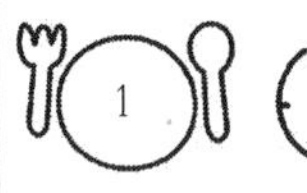 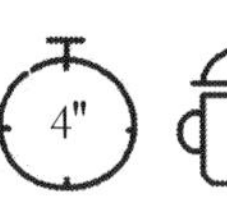 

12.8 Blueberry Smoothie

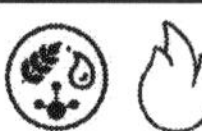  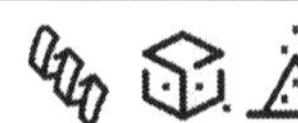 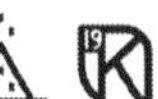

per serving	171 Cal	5.7g	17.4g	14.1g	13.4g	450 mg

- Fresh or frozen blueberries – ½ cup
- Oats – ¼ cup
- Coconut milk – ½ cup
- Lemon zest – ½ tsp.
- Vanilla powder – 1 tsp.

1. In a blender or food processor, combine or process all ingredients until completely smooth.

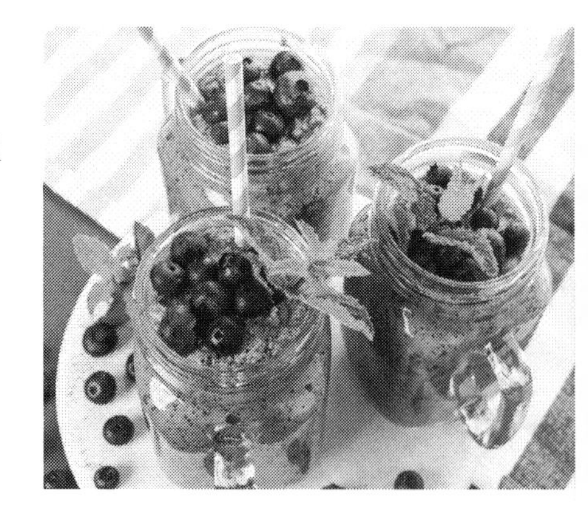

Storage:
For a maximum of three months, you can keep smoothies or their components in the freezer.

 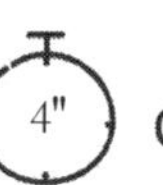 

1 | 4" | 0"

12.9 Green Kiwi Smoothie

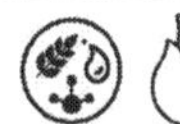 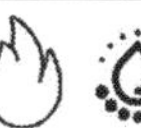 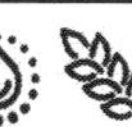 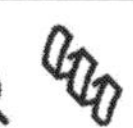 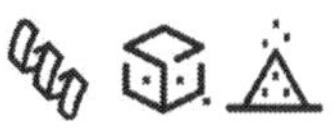 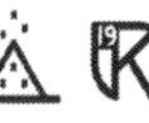

per serving	184 Cal	0.7g	45.3g	3g	33.4g		450 mg

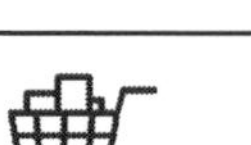

- 8 tbsp, mashed unripe banana
- ½ tsp Olive oil
- 4 eggs

1. In a blender or food processor, combine or process all ingredients until completely smooth.

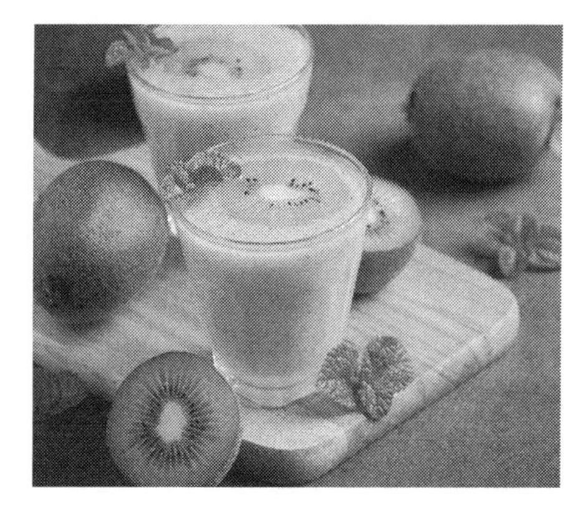

Storage:
For a maximum of three months, you can keep smoothies or their components in the freezer.

 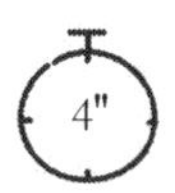 

1 | 4" | 0"

12.10 Orange Carrot Juice

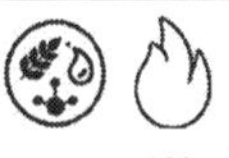  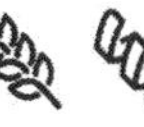 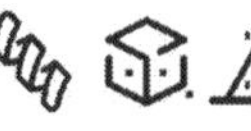 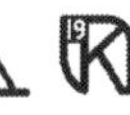

per serving	198 Cal	2.1g	22g	23.4g	14g		599 mg

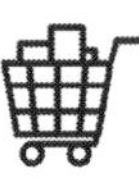

- Freshly squeezed carrot juice – ½ cup
- Freshly squeezed orange juice – ½ cup
- Protein powder- 1 scoop

1. In a blender or food processor, combine or process all ingredients until completely smooth.

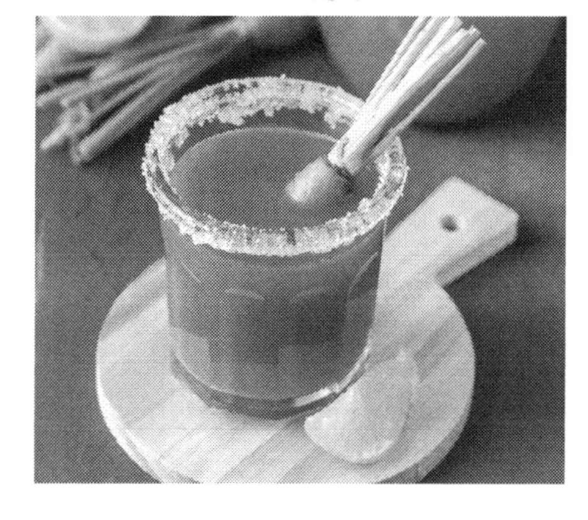

Storage:
For a maximum of three months, you can keep smoothies or their components in the freezer.

CHAPTER 13

DESSERTS RECIPES

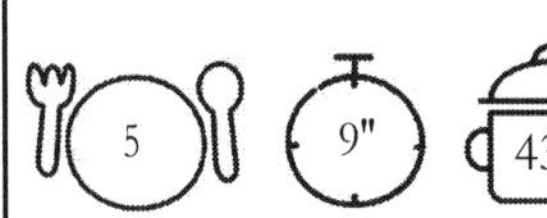

13.1 Strawberry Crisp

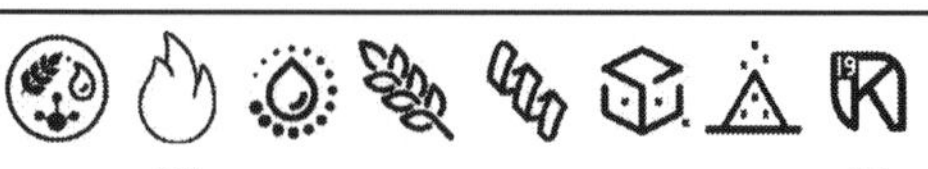

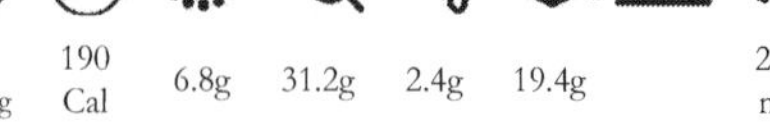

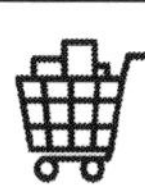

Topping

- Vegan butter or lactose-free butter – 2 tbsp.
- Oat flour – 1/3 cup
- Cinnamon, ground – ¼ tsp
- Salt, 1/8 teaspoon
- Old-fashioned rolled oats, 1/3 cup (gluten free if necessary)
- Brown sugar, 1/3 cup

When filling:

- Strawberries – 3 cups
- Corn starch or tapioca starch, 1 tbsp
- Cane sugar- 2 tbsp.
- Salt, a pinch
- Vanilla extract, 1 tsp.

1. Set the oven's temperature to 350 degrees Fahrenheit. Any form of 8 or 9-inch glass baking dish, sprayed with cooking oil spray.
2. The quartered strawberries, corn or tapioca starch (also known as tapioca flour), sugar, salt, and vanilla essence go into the filling. Scoop into the baking dish after stirring the ingredients together.
3. In a medium bowl, combine the brown sugar, oat flour, cinnamon, and salt to make the topping. Cut the butter into the sugar mixture with forks, a pastry cutter, or your fingertips until pea-sized lumps form. Sprinkle the topping over the strawberry filling after incorporating the oats.
4. Bake for 40 to 45 minutes, or until the topping is just beginning to turn brown and the strawberries are bubbling, in the oven. Before serving, take the food out of the oven and let it cool slightly on a wire rack.

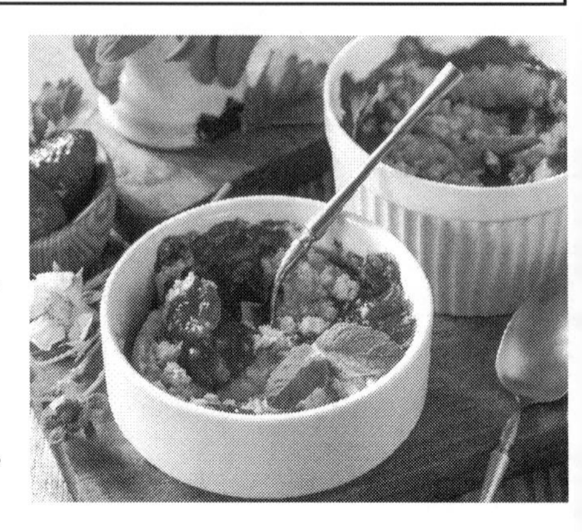

Storage:
For up to five days, keep leftovers covered in the refrigerator.

 5 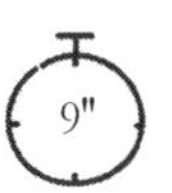 9"  55"

13.2 Fudgesicles

 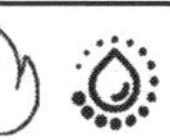 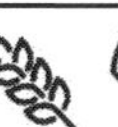 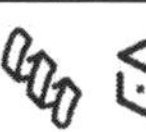 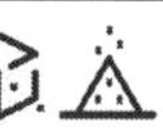 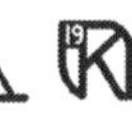

per serving	298 Cal	24.6g	14.4g	2.3g	10.4g		38 mg

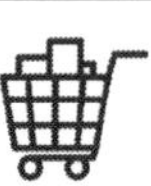

- Pure vanilla extract, 2 tsp.
- Cocoa powder, dark - 1/2 cup
- Maple syrup - 1/3 cup
- Coconut milk, chilled – 2 cups

1. Blend all the ingredients together in a blender until they are completely smooth.
2. In a popsicle mold, pour the mixture.
3. Freeze overnight or for at least four hours.

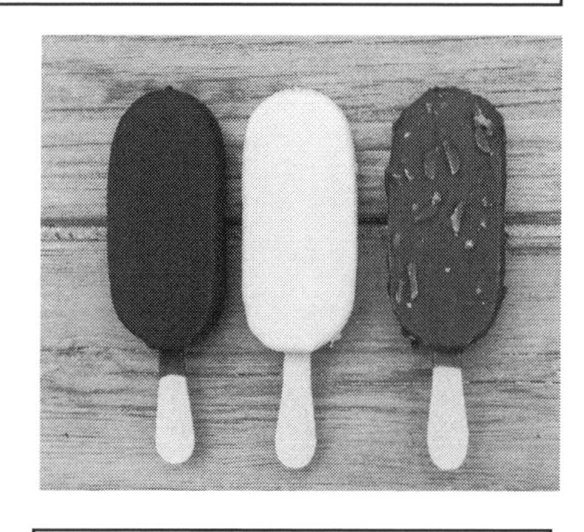

Storage:
For up to three months, freeze.

 15 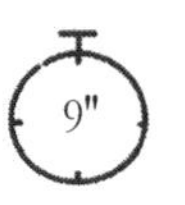 9"  55"

13.3 Cocoa Crinkle Cookies

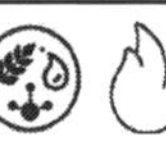  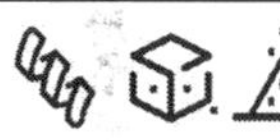 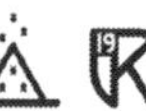 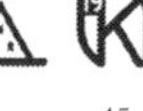

per serving	95 Cal	3.6g	15.4g	1.2g	8.4g		45 mg

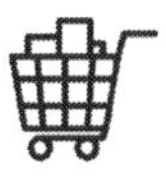

- Sugar, granulated – 1 cup
- Baking powder – 1 tbsp.
- Pinch salt
- Coconut oil, 1/3 cup
- Unsweetened cocoa powder, 1/3 cup
- Beaten eggs - 2
- Vanilla extract, 1 teaspoon
- Coconut flour -1 ¼ cups

1. Salt, baking soda, cocoa powder, and flour should be sifted into a medium basin and thoroughly combined.
2. Whisk the sugar and canola oil together in a large bowl. It will resemble damp sand somewhat. Stir in the eggs and vanilla after adding them. The flour mixture should be added gradually while being thoroughly blended. The texture will resemble thick brownie batter in some ways.
3. Refrigerate the dough with a cover for at least six hours.
4. Set the oven at 350 degrees Fahrenheit after the dough has thoroughly chilled. Using parchment paper, line a sizable cookie sheet. The powdered sugar should be put in a small basin.
5. Take the dough out of the fridge. This dough has a tendency to become a little sticky, especially as it warms up. Quick thinking is essential. To assist stop the dough from sticking to my hands, Each ball should be well coated in powdered sugar. On the prepared baking sheet, arrange the covered dough balls at least 2 inches apart from one another.
6. The tops should be cracked and no longer moist after baking for 11 to 13 minutes. There will still be some softness inside. After taking the cookies out of the oven, let them cool on the cookie sheet for two to three minutes. The cookies should then be moved to a wire rack to cool until room temperature. Serve.

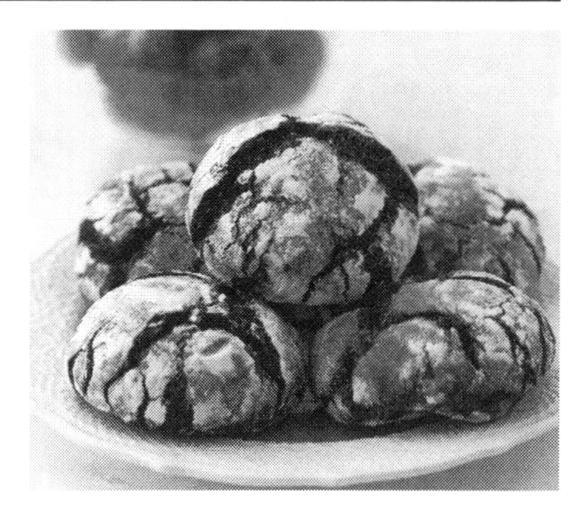

Storage:
Cookies can be kept for up to 5 days after they have totally cooled down. For up to three months, freeze.

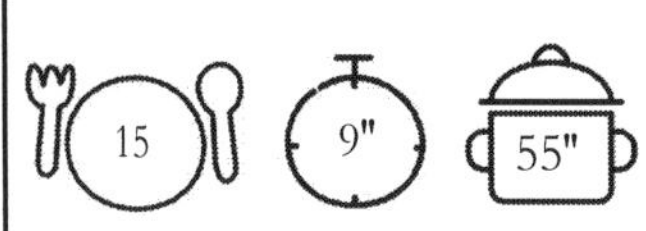

15 | 9" | 55"

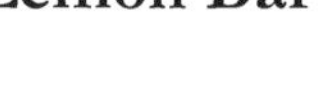

13.4 Lemon Bar

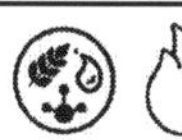 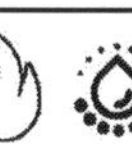 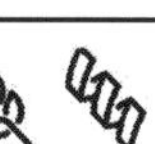 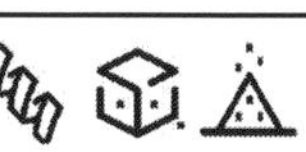

per serving | 149 Cal | 7.4g | 18.5g | 2.4g | 6.4g | 28 mg

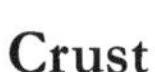

Crust

- Gluten-free Baking Flour- 1 ½ cups
- Granulated sugar, ½ cup
- Unsalted butter – ½ cup
- Water, 3 tbsp,

Citrus Topping

- Gluten-Free Baking Flour, 1/4 cup
- Lightly beaten eggs - 4
- Freshly squeezed lemon juice in a half cup (about 3 lemons)
- Granulated sugar, 1 1/2 cups

1. Set the oven to 350°F. A 9-inch baking pan should be butter-greased or lined with parchment paper.
2. To make the crust: Combine 1 1/2 cups flour and 1/2 cup sugar in a medium bowl. Crumble the butter into the flour mixture using a pastry blender. Then combine in 3 tbsp, of water. (Occasionally, I'll pulse the crust ingredients in a food processor until they resemble coarse crumbs.) In the bottom of the greased pan, press the mixture.
3. Bake crust for 20 to 22 minutes, or until firm and somewhat puffy. (Note: Unlike crusts made with wheat, gluten-free crusts don't often brown.
4. While the crust is baking, prepare the lemon topping by thoroughly combining the eggs, lemon juice, 1 12 cups sugar, and 1/4 cup flour. Pour over the baked crust uniformly.
5. Bake an additional 20 to 25 minutes, or until the lemon topping is set. (To determine if the middle still jiggles, I put on an oven mitt and lightly shake the pan.) After baking, remove the bars and let them cool for about two hours to room temperature.
6. Sprinkle some optional powdered sugar on top to garnish. Serve after cutting into 16 pieces.

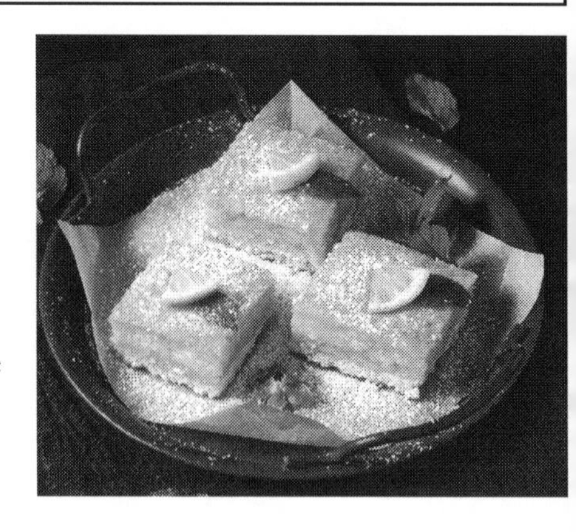

Storage:
For up to a week, cover and chill any remaining bars.

1 | 2" | 2"

13.5 Mug Cake

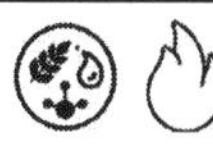   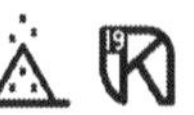

per serving | 214 Cal | 11.4g | 30.3g | 1.8g | 14g | 360 mg

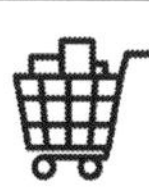

- Baking powder – ½ tsp.
- Cocoa - 2 tbsp..
- Boil water - 3 tbsp.
- Oil - 1 1/2 tbsp,
- Tapioca flour - 1/9 cup
- Pinch of salt, fine
- Pure maple syrup -2 1/2 tsp.
- Gluten-free flour -2 tbsp.

1. In a small bowl, combine the cocoa and the boiling water. Whisk in the oil and maple syrup until smooth.
2. Tapioca flour should be added and whisked in until completely smooth. Even though it will initially appear to be an oily mess, adding the tapioca flour before the brown rice flour makes the batter smoother in the end.
3. Whisk until smooth before adding the brown rice flour (or other gluten-free wholegrain flour of your choice; see notes). Salt and baking powder are then added and thoroughly combined.
4. Set the oven's temperature to 180 C (356 F). Pour the mixture into a ceramic baking dish that can be used in an oven (I use a ceramic tiny casserole dish with a 1 1/2 cup capacity).
5. The cake should be baked for 15 to 20 minutes. You can let some of the fudgy chunks cook until they are fully cooked. Serve.

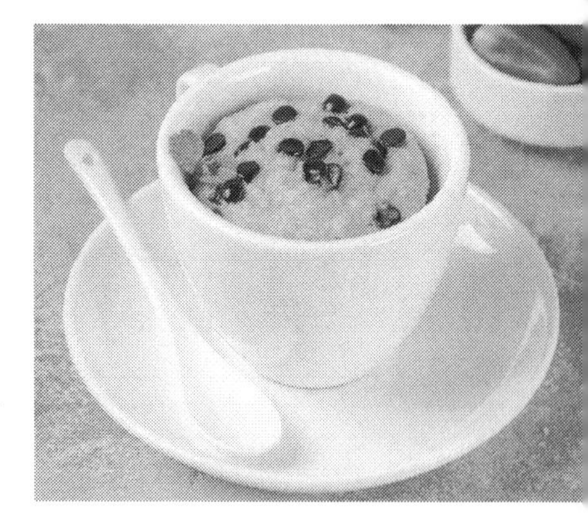

Storage:
For up to three months, freeze.

 37 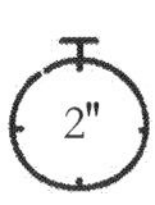 2"  2"

13.6 Chocolate Peanut Butter

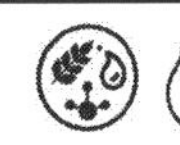 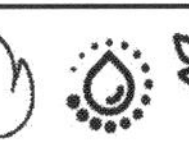 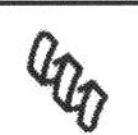 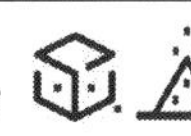 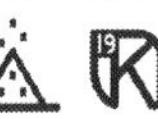 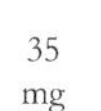

per serving | 42 Cal | 3.6g | 1.6g | 1.4g | 0.5g | 35 mg

- Margarine – ¼ cup
- Semi-sweet chocolate – 8 ounce
- Peanut butter- 9 ounces
- Confectioner's sugar - 1 & 3/4 cup
- Gluten-free (low-FODMAP) crisped rice cereal -1 & 1/4 cup

1. In a large mixing bowl of a stand mixer, combine vegan butter, peanut butter, and sugar. Beat until smooth.
2. Rice grain should be added, then very slowly stirred in with a flat paddle or by hand
3. Put the bowl in the fridge and let it become cold there (About 45 minutes)
4. A baking sheet should be prepared using parchment or wax paper.
5. Form into 1-inch balls with a tiny cookie scoop or melon baller, then set on a baking sheet.
6. Place the balls in the refrigerator for a minimum of 12 hours.
7. Melt chocolate in a double boiler.
8. Replace the balls on the cookie sheet and refrigerate once more until serving after dipping them in the chocolate.
9. Most effective when slightly cold.

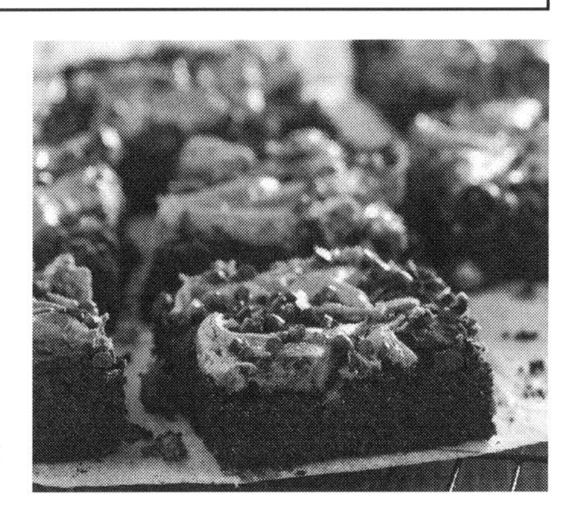

Storage:
For up to three months, freeze.

 23 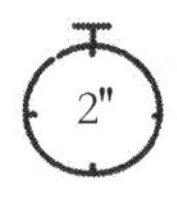 2" 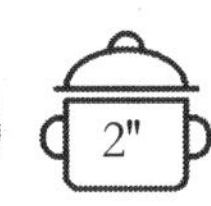 2"

13.7 Peanut Butter Cookies

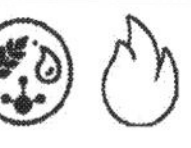  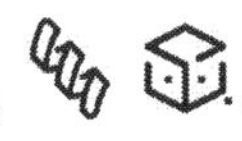 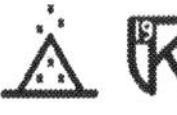 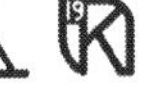

per serving | 91 Cal | 5.4g | 8g | 3.4g | 6.5g | 10 mg

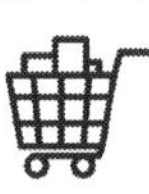

- Brown sugar, 1 cup
- Natural peanut butter, 1 cup
- Ground flaxseed – 1 tbsp.

1. Set the oven to 350°F.
2. Combine the flax with 3 tbsp water in a small bowl. Give it five minutes to sit.
3. In a big basin, thoroughly combine all ingredients. To create 1 cookie, roll about 1 tbsp of dough into a ball and set on baking sheet. To flatten, use a fork to gently press down. Add optional toppings on top.
4. Bake for 10 minutes, or until the edges are just starting to brown. Allow the pan to cool for 5 minutes. When taken out of the oven, cookies are quite soft, but as they cool, they become slightly harder.

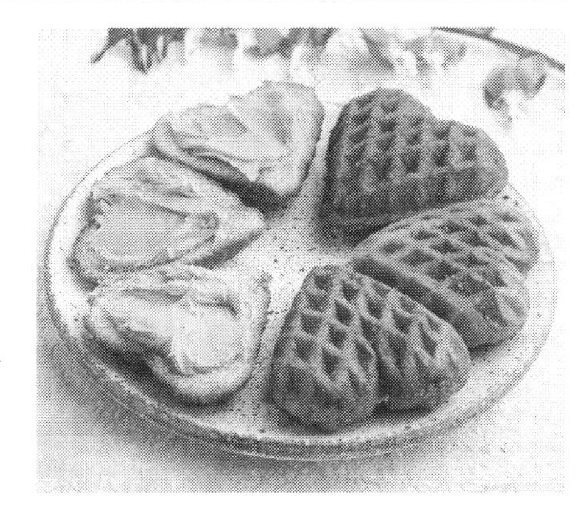

Storage:
For up to three months, freeze.

 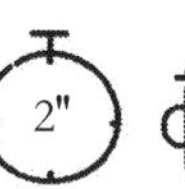 

13.8 Blueberry lemon mug cake

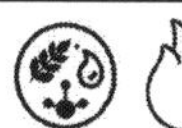 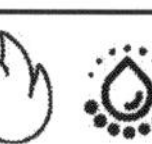 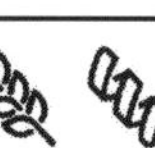 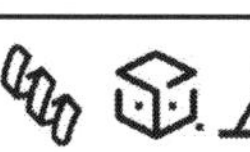 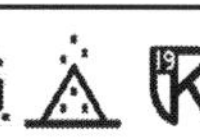

per serving	501 Cal	15.7g	75.8g	1.7g	2.3g	176 mg

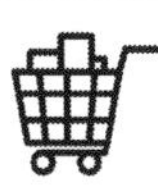

- Pure vanilla extract, 2 tsp
- Granulated sugar, 2 tbsp
- Salt, a pinch
- Coconut milk, 1/2 cup
- Melted unsalted butter- 1 tbsp.
- Baking powder- ¼ tsp
- Lemon zest – 1tsp
- Blueberries,- ¼ cup
- All-purpose flour -1/2 cup

1. Get a 12-ounce mug for yourself. Whisk together the salt, baking powder, sugar, and flour.
2. Whisk once more before adding the milk, butter, vanilla, and lemon zest.
3. Fold the blueberries in with a spoon or fork after adding them.
4. Your mug cake should be heated in the microwave until just done (about 2ish minutes depending on your microwave).

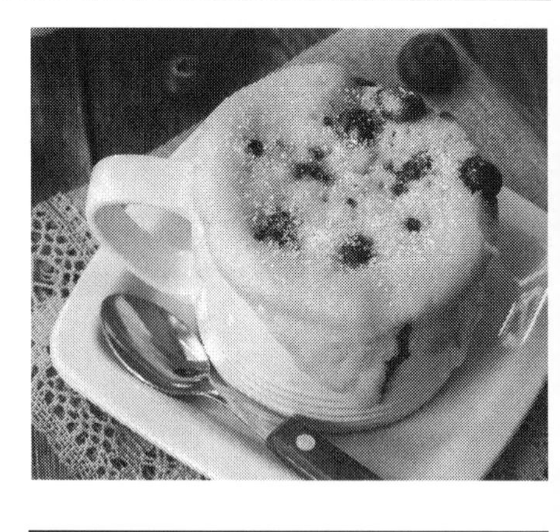

Storage:
Cookies can be frozen for three weeks and can be stored at room temperature for three days.

 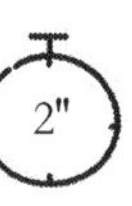 

13.9 Almond Thumbprint Cookies

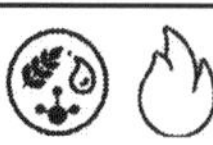 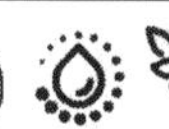 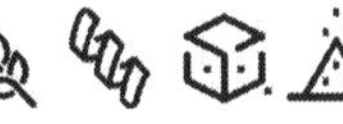 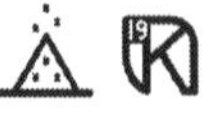

per serving	92 Cal	7.3g	5.8g	1.7g	2.3g	1 mg

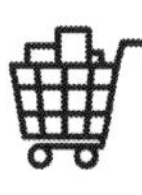

- Almond flour - 1 cup
- Sea salt - 1/8 teaspoon
- Unsalted butter 3-1/2 tbsp.
- Granulated sugar – 3 tablespoon
- Vanilla extract, 1/2 teaspoon.

1. Set the oven to 350°F. Use parchment paper to cover a baking sheet.
2. Place all ingredients in the bowl of an electric mixer minus and blend on medium speed until a doughy mixture develops (or mix by hand).
3. Scoop dough by the heaping teaspoon and form it into 1 1/4-inch balls. Place on baking sheet and space 1 1/2 to 2 inches apart. Each dough ball needs a thumbprint imprint in the middle.
4. Bake the cookies for 9 to 12 minutes, or until the edges feel just set. Cookies won't brown all that much.
5. Take the cookies out of the oven and let them cool for 10 minutes on the baking sheet. Before serving, move them to a rack to thoroughly cool.

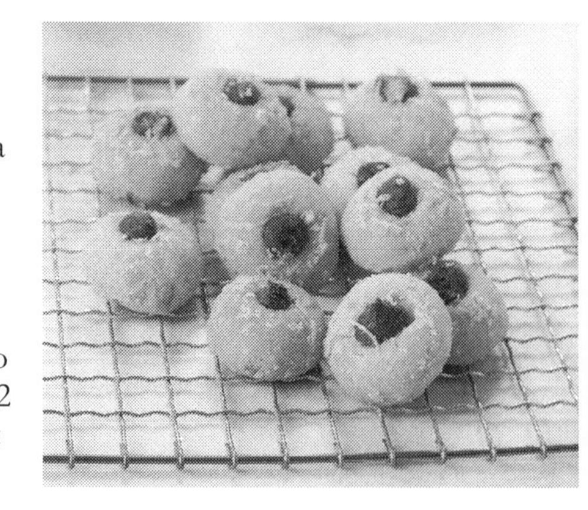

Storage:
Cookies can be frozen for three weeks and can be stored at room temperature for three days.

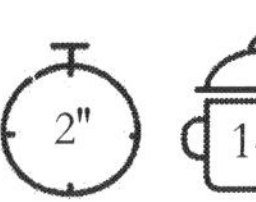

13.10 Orange-Pecan Cookies

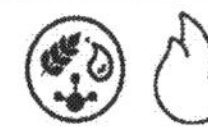 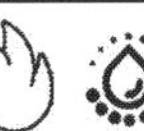 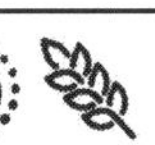 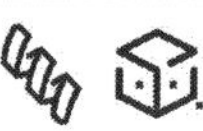  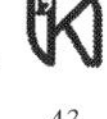

per serving	73 Cal	5.4g	6.1g	1.1g	5.2g	43 mg

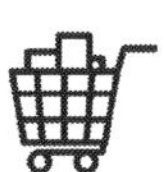

- Pecans, 2 cups
- Sugar -2/3 cup
- Egg whites - 2
- Orange's zest- 1
- Sea salt – ½ tsp.
- Cooking spray

1. Set the oven to 350°F. Pecans should be spread out on a big baking sheet with a rim and baked for 7 to 8 minutes, stirring them approximately halfway through, until aromatic and lightly toasted. Complete cooling.
2. Place the sugar in the bowl of a food processor with a metal blade and add the cooled pecans (they must be cooled or they will become pasty). Once finely chopped with a chunky, slightly sandy texture, pulse several times.
3. Combine egg whites, orange zest, extracts, and salt in a big bowl. Stir the pecan mixture in before adding it. Refrigerate for 90 to 2 hours, or until totally cold.
4. Set the racks in the upper and lower thirds of the oven and preheat it to 350°F. Cooking spray or shortening should be used to oil two baking sheets of parchment paper. Place heaping teaspoons of batter about 2 inches apart on parchment. Expect to receive 28 to 30 cookies.
5. Bake for 13 to 15 minutes, or until cookies are puffy and barely set in the center. About halfway through, switch the baking sheets' up-down-back positions. After five minutes of cooling on the baking sheets, move to a rack to finish cooling.

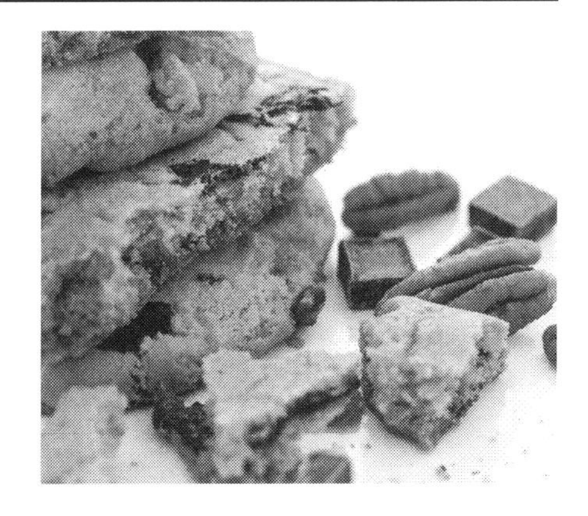

Storage:
For up to three months, freeze.

CHAPTER 14

15-DAY MEAL PLAN TO RESET YOUR BODY

Days	Breakfast	Lunch	Dinner	Dessert
1	Breakfast Egg Muffins	Grilled Pork Chops with Lemon & Sage	Kale Quinoa	Peanut Butter Cookies
2	Quinoa Porridge	Broccoli Feta Soup	Caramelized Salmon	Chocolate Peanut Butter
3		Greek Grilled Chicken	Chicken Zucchini Soup	Mug Cake
4	Banana Egg Pancakes	Quick Shrimp Stir Fry	Maple Mustard Baked Chicken	Fudgesicles
5	Egg muffins with quinoa	Chili con carne		Cocoa Crinkle Cookies
6	Baked Eggs in Kale and Tomato	Olive Oil Roasted Eggplant with Lemon	Herb-Roasted Salmon	Strawberry Crisp
7	Buckwheat Breakfast Porridge	Maple Mustard Baked Chicken	Lemon Herb Quinoa	Lemon Bar
8	Tomato Omelet	Sesame Green Beans	Grilled Pork Chops with Lemon & Sage	Peanut Butter Cookies
9	Eggs in Cloud	Greek Grilled Chicken	Roasted Squash Soup	Chocolate Peanut Butter
10	Flaxseed Flour Muffins		Chili con carne	Mug Cake
11	Peppers Scrambled Eggs	Spicy Grilled Shrimp		Fudgesicles
12	Overnight Oats	Skillet Kale with Lemon	Maple Mustard Baked Chicken	Cocoa Crinkle Cookies
13	Tomato Omelet	Grilled Pork Chops with Lemon & Sage	Sautéed Yellow Squash	Orange-Pecan Cookies
14	Eggs in Cloud	Zucchini Soup	Greek Grilled Chicken	Almond Thumbprint Cookies
15	Flaxseed Flour Muffins	Chili con carne	Kale Quinoa	Blueberry lemon mug cake

CHAPTER 15

10 WEEKS MEAL PLAN TO STAY HEALTHY LONGER

I prepared a meal plan for 10 weeks which is about 2 1/2 months. Repeating this meal plan 5-6 times throughout the year, starting from the first week after the tenth, you will have concluded your annual nutrition plan. To ensure the habit of this diet and the results, we recommend applying it for 3 years, consequently for a total of 1000 days.

Week 1

Days	Breakfast	Lunch	Dinner	Dessert
1	Breakfast Egg Muffins	Grilled Pork Chops with Lemon & Sage	Kale Quinoa	Peanut Butter Cookies
2	Quinoa Porridge	Broccoli Feta Soup	Caramelized Salmon	Chocolate Peanut Butter
3		Greek Grilled Chicken	Chicken Zucchini Soup	Mug Cake
4	Banana Egg Pancakes	Quick Shrimp Stir Fry	Maple Mustard Baked Chicken	Fudgesicles
5	Egg muffins with quinoa	Chili con carne		Cocoa Crinkle Cookies
6	Baked Eggs in Kale and Tomato	Olive Oil Roasted Eggplant with Lemon	Herb-Roasted Salmon	Strawberry Crisp
7	Buckwheat Breakfast Porridge	Maple Mustard Baked Chicken	Lemon Herb Quinoa	Lemon Bar

Week 2

Days	Breakfast	Lunch	Dinner	Dessert
1	Eggs in Cloud	Greek Grilled Chicken	Roasted Squash Soup	Chocolate Peanut Butter
2	Flaxseed Flour Muffins		Chili con carne	Mug Cake
3	Peppers Scrambled Eggs	Spicy Grilled Shrimp		Fudgesicles
4	Overnight Oats	Skillet Kale with Lemon	Maple Mustard Baked Chicken	Cocoa Crinkle Cookies
5	Tomato Omelet	Grilled Pork Chops with Lemon & Sage	Sautéed Yellow Squash	Orange-Pecan Cookies
6	Eggs in Cloud	Zucchini Soup	Greek Grilled Chicken	Almond Thumbprint Cookies
7	Flaxseed Flour Muffins	Maple Mustard Baked Chicken	Lemon Herb Quinoa	Lemon Bar

Week 3

Days	Breakfast	Lunch	Dinner	Dessert
1	Quinoa Porridge	Broccoli Feta Soup	Caramelized Salmon	Chocolate Peanut Butter
2		Greek Grilled Chicken	Chicken Zucchini Soup	Mug Cake
3	Banana Egg Pancakes	Quick Shrimp Stir Fry	Maple Mustard Baked Chicken	Fudgesicles
4	Egg muffins with quinoa	Chili con carne		Cocoa Crinkle Cookies
5	Baked Eggs in Kale and Tomato	Olive Oil Roasted Eggplant with Lemon	Herb-Roasted Salmon	Strawberry Crisp
6	Buckwheat Breakfast Porridge	Maple Mustard Baked Chicken	Lemon Herb Quinoa	Lemon Bar
7	Tomato Omelet	Sesame Green Beans	Grilled Pork Chops with Lemon & Sage	Peanut Butter Cookies

Week 4

Days	Breakfast	Lunch	Dinner	Dessert
1	Banana Egg Pancakes	Quick Shrimp Stir Fry	Maple Mustard Baked Chicken	Fudgesicles
2	Egg muffins with quinoa	Chili con carne		Cocoa Crinkle Cookies
3	Baked Eggs in Kale and Tomato	Olive Oil Roasted Eggplant with Lemon	Herb-Roasted Salmon	Strawberry Crisp
4	Buckwheat Breakfast Porridge	Maple Mustard Baked Chicken	Lemon Herb Quinoa	Lemon Bar
5	Tomato Omelet	Sesame Green Beans	Grilled Pork Chops with Lemon & Sage	Peanut Butter Cookies
6	Eggs in Cloud	Greek Grilled Chicken	Roasted Squash Soup	Chocolate Peanut Butter
7	Flaxseed Flour Muffins		Chili con carne	Mug Cake

Week 5

Days	Breakfast	Lunch	Dinner	Dessert
1	Peppers Scrambled Eggs	Spicy Grilled Shrimp		Fudgesicles
2	Overnight Oats	Skillet Kale with Lemon	Maple Mustard Baked Chicken	Cocoa Crinkle Cookies
3	Tomato Omelet	Grilled Pork Chops with Lemon & Sage	Sautéed Yellow Squash	Orange-Pecan Cookies
4	Eggs in Cloud	Zucchini Soup	Greek Grilled Chicken	Almond Thumbprint Cookies
5	Flaxseed Flour Muffins	Chili con carne	Kale Quinoa	Blueberry lemon mug cake
6	Peppers Scrambled Eggs	Spicy Grilled Shrimp		Fudgesicles
7	Overnight Oats	Skillet Kale with Lemon	Maple Mustard Baked Chicken	Cocoa Crinkle Cookies

Week 6

Days	Breakfast	Lunch	Dinner	Dessert
1	Baked Eggs in Kale and Tomato	Olive Oil Roasted Eggplant with Lemon	Herb-Roasted Salmon	Strawberry Crisp
2	Buckwheat Breakfast Porridge	Maple Mustard Baked Chicken	Lemon Herb Quinoa	Lemon Bar
3	Tomato Omelet	Sesame Green Beans	Grilled Pork Chops with Lemon & Sage	Peanut Butter Cookies
4	Baked Eggs in Kale and Tomato	Olive Oil Roasted Eggplant with Lemon	Herb-Roasted Salmon	Strawberry Crisp
5	Flaxseed Flour Muffins	Chili con carne	Kale Quinoa	Blueberry lemon mug cake
6	Peppers Scrambled Eggs	Spicy Grilled Shrimp		Fudgesicles
7	Overnight Oats	Skillet Kale with Lemon	Maple Mustard Baked Chicken	Cocoa Crinkle Cookies

Week 7

Days	Breakfast	Lunch	Dinner	Dessert
1	Baked Eggs in Kale and Tomato	Olive Oil Roasted Eggplant with Lemon	Herb-Roasted Salmon	Strawberry Crisp
2	Buckwheat Breakfast Porridge	Maple Mustard Baked Chicken	Lemon Herb Quinoa	Lemon Bar
3	Tomato Omelet	Sesame Green Beans	Grilled Pork Chops with Lemon & Sage	Peanut Butter Cookies
4	Baked Eggs in Kale and Tomato	Olive Oil Roasted Eggplant with Lemon	Herb-Roasted Salmon	Strawberry Crisp
5	Flaxseed Flour Muffins	Chili con carne	Kale Quinoa	Blueberry lemon mug cake
6	Peppers Scrambled Eggs	Spicy Grilled Shrimp	Tuscan Salmon	Fudgesicles
7	Overnight Oats	Skillet Kale with Lemon	Maple Mustard Baked Chicken	Cocoa Crinkle Cookies

Week 8

Days	Breakfast	Lunch	Dinner	Dessert
1	Baked Eggs in Kale and Tomato	Olive Oil Roasted Eggplant with Lemon	Herb-Roasted Salmon	Strawberry Crisp
2	Buckwheat Breakfast Porridge	Maple Mustard Baked Chicken	Lemon Herb Quinoa	Lemon Bar
3	Tomato Omelet	Sesame Green Beans	Grilled Pork Chops with Lemon & Sage	Peanut Butter Cookies
4	Baked Eggs in Kale and Tomato	Olive Oil Roasted Eggplant with Lemon	Herb-Roasted Salmon	Strawberry Crisp
5	Flaxseed Flour Muffins	Chili con carne	Kale Quinoa	Blueberry lemon mug cake
6	Peppers Scrambled Eggs	Chicken Fajitas	Quick Korean Beef	Fudgesicles
7	Overnight Oats	Tandoori Chicken	Maple Mustard Baked Chicken	Cocoa Crinkle Cookies

Week 9

Days	Breakfast	Lunch	Dinner	Dessert
1	Sesame Breakfast Pudding	Olive Oil Roasted Eggplant with Lemon	Herb-Roasted Salmon	Strawberry Crisp
2	Buckwheat Breakfast Porridge	Maple Mustard Baked Chicken	Lemon Herb Quinoa	Lemon Bar
3	Overnight Oats	Sesame Green Beans	Grilled Pork Chops with Lemon & Sage	Peanut Butter Cookies
4	Baked Eggs in Kale and Tomato	Olive Oil Roasted Eggplant with Lemon	Herb-Roasted Salmon	Strawberry Crisp
5	Flaxseed Flour Muffins	Easy Kale Salad	Roasted Squash Soup	Blueberry lemon mug cake
6	Peppers Scrambled Eggs	Tuscan Salmon	Chicken Fajitas	Fudgesicles
7	Overnight Oats	Skillet Kale with Lemon	Maple Mustard Baked Chicken	Cocoa Crinkle Cookies

Week 10

Days	Breakfast	Lunch	Dinner	Dessert
1	Baked Eggs in Kale and Tomato	Olive Oil Roasted Eggplant with Lemon	Herb-Roasted Salmon	Strawberry Crisp
2	Buckwheat Breakfast Porridge	Maple Mustard Baked Chicken	Lemon Herb Quinoa	Lemon Bar
3	Tomato Omelet	Sesame Green Beans	Grilled Pork Chops with Lemon & Sage	Peanut Butter Cookies
4	Baked Eggs in Kale and Tomato	Olive Oil Roasted Eggplant with Lemon	Herb-Roasted Salmon	Strawberry Crisp
5	Flaxseed Flour Muffins	Chili con carne	Kale Quinoa	Blueberry lemon mug cake
6	Peppers Scrambled Eggs	Spicy Grilled Shrimp	Quick Korean Beef	Fudgesicles
7	Overnight Oats	Skillet Kale with Lemon	Maple Mustard Baked Chicken	Cocoa Crinkle Cookies

CHAPTER 16

MEASUREMENT CONVERSION CHART

16.1 Volume Equivalents (Dry)

Imperial	Mertic (Approximate)
1/8 teaspoon	0.5 mL
1/4 teaspoon	1 mL
1/2 teaspoon	2 mL
3/4 teaspoon	4 mL
1 teaspoon	5 mL
1 tablespoon	15 mL
1/4 cup	59 mL
1/2 cup	118 mL
3/4 cup	177 mL
1 cup	235 mL
2 cups	475 mL
3 cups	700 mL
4 cups	1 L

16.2 Temperature Equivalents

Fahrenheit (F)	Mertic (Approximate)
225 °F	107 °C
250 °F	120 °C
275 °F	135 °C
300 °F	150 °C
325 °F	160 °C
350 °F	180 °C
375 °F	190 °C
400 °F	205 °C
425 °F	220 °C
450 °F	235 °C
475 °F	245 °C
500 °F	260 °C

16.3 Volume Equivalents (Liquid)

US STANDARD	US STANDARD (Ounces)	Mertic (Approximate)
2 tablespoons	1 fl. oz.	30 mL
1/4 cup	2 fl. oz.	60 mL
1/2 cup	4 fl. oz.	120 mL
1 cup	8 fl. oz.	240 mL
1 1/2 cup	12 fl. oz.	355 mL
2 cups or 1 pint	16 fl. oz.	475 mL
4 cups or 1 quart	32 fl. oz.	1 L
1 gallon	128 fl. oz.	4 L

16.4 Weight Equivalents

US STANDARD	Mertic (Approximate)
1 ounce	28 g
2 ounces	57 g
5 ounces	142 g
10 ounces	284 g
15 ounces	425 g
16 ounces (1 pound)	455 g
1.5 pounds	680 g
2 pounds	907 g

CONCLUSION

For those with IBS, a low-FODMAP diet may significantly reduce their symptoms.

But not everyone with IBS reacts to the diet, and it includes a three-stage approach that could take up to 8 weeks to yield results.

FODMAPs are prebiotics that promote gut health, so unless you really need them, this diet can be more harmful than helpful. Additionally, foods high in FODMAP are important nutritional sources of vitamins and minerals.

However, if you have IBS, this diet may significantly enhance your quality of life.

A three-step diet called a FODMAP diet is used to assist treat irritable bowel syndrome, which has been medically diagnosed (IBS). The symptoms of IBS, which is a fairly prevalent gastrointestinal condition, include stomach pain, bloating, wind (farting), and changes in bowel habits (diarrhea, constipation or both).

The diet's objectives are to:

Find out which foods and FODMAPs you can tolerate, as well as which ones make your IBS symptoms worse. Understanding this will make it easier for you to stick to a long-term diet that only restricts the items that make your IBS symptoms worse and is more nutritionally balanced.

Check to see if your IBS symptoms are affected by FODMAPs. Not every IBS patient will benefit from a low FODMAP diet. It is crucial to know if you fall into the category of the 34 of IBS sufferers who experience symptom improvement on the diet or the 14 of IBS sufferers who do not and must consequently investigate other IBS therapy.

BONUS: Scanning the following QR code will take you to a web page where you can access 3 fantastic bonuses after leaving your email contact: 3 mobile apps for Android and iOS to assist you in your nutrition and cooking.

LINK: https://BookHip.com/ZBFKSRG

Made in the USA
Monee, IL
29 November 2022

99778c21-d957-4b0c-a8b9-13b7ee73c366R01